Multiple Sclerosis

Smiling & Hurting

Dorothy M. Mitchell

chipmunkapublishing

the mental health publisher

Dorothy M. Mitchell

Published by
Chipmunkapublishing
PO Box 6872
Brentwood
Essex CM13 1ZT
United Kingdom

http://www.chipmunkapublishing.com

Edited by Lucy Lythgoe

ISBN   978-1-84991-725-4

Chipmunkapublishing   gratefully   acknowledge   the
support of Arts Council England.

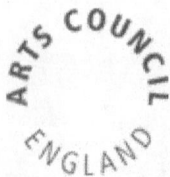

ARTS COUNCIL
ENGLAND

CHAPTER ONE

CHILDHOOD IN YORKSHIRE

I was born in a small Yorkshire village just before the Second World War. I was born blind in my left eye, something to do with the optic nerve not forming properly I believe. I can't say I ever miss it for they do say: "what you have never had you don't miss" , but I remember as a child I used to drive myself mad trying to see the left side of my nose when I looked cross-eyed down the front of my nose, it was easy to see the right side but I could never see the left.

Mum used to tell the tale of me having both eyes out when I was a baby when a consultant in that particular field, attempted to restore the sight, an operation done by a German specialist! She used to say my eyes looked like two pieces of liver after the op for ages afterwards, but I was still blind in my left eye. She also said I cried a great deal during that time. I don't remember it though; I have no recollection at all, of that particular incident. Perhaps that's a good thing! Looking back it must have been traumatic for Mum! I say this because my youngest son David suffered night colic when he was a young baby; night after night he screamed pulling his little legs up to his chest. Gripe water and being cuddled were his only comfort. These colic attacks finally abated when he was about 6 months old, by that time both his dad and I were worn out. I don't think gripe water is available now, new, supposedly better products taking its place. All I know is that at the time gripe water was my much needed friend, and David's soothing balm.

What I do remember about my fearful school days though, was the horrible glasses I had to wear. They featured in my life from the age of two years old. They had round lenses in a frame with curly sides that used to rub my ears sore. I had a pronounced squint in my blind eye and somehow the lens in the glasses acted like a magnet to prevent my eye from turning into the corner.

I was the eldest of three children. Mum used to talk about a baby born before me. She was premature and weighed only one pound. She died at the age of one week. Mum said Maureen, that was the baby's name, would have easily fitted into a pint pot. Looking back to that time it must have hurt Mum a great deal. I never did find where the baby had been buried, it wasn't talked about, another thing that I found strange when my brother and sister were growing up. Mum never encouraged us to cuddle each other, it simply wasn't done. In fact mum never told me she loved me until shortly before her death at the age of 89 years. I had sworn to myself years earlier, that if I got married and had kids they would be told they were loved. Perhaps there was some reason for this in Mum's own childhood. I am not saying we were badly treated, on the contrary we were well looked after, but there was just something that made Mum hold back on showing affection!

When I was two years old my brother Brian was born followed three years later by Sandra my sister. I remember vividly Brian and myself going into the Air Raid shelter Dad had built in our garden. It was dark and cold. The dreaded sirens had just gone off telling us that there was another attack from enemy planes, coming over the night sky. Mum was on the doorstep holding newly born baby Sandra. We all rushed into the dark shelter to the fearful drone of aircraft overhead , with just a few candles for light, care being taken not to show the smallest chink of light at all. If you did, you heard the Air raid Warden shout, "PUT THAT BLOODY

LIGHT OUT." If you have ever watched DAD'S ARMY, on TV then you will know exactly what I mean!

This happened on a regular basis, and it was horrible. We never had a bomb drop on our village although there was an underground aerodrome close by, and according to what I have been told since, the enemy were looking for the place for ages. They never did find it.   I can see Mum now sweeping shrapnel from our garden path after an air raid!

Being inside the Anderson shelter during an Air raid was very scary. The loud noise of aircraft overhead, the sound of bombs whistling down was frightening. I was about five years old at the time, I didn't understand the terrible implications of what was going on but I knew it was pretty bad.

I started school at the age of three, and from the very first day I hated it. We had to take our gasmasks to school. I couldn't bear the smell of it when we had to practice wearing them. Having my face in the thing was horrible. It smelled of something nasty, all rubbery. Anyway, it was frightening. I felt I couldn't breathe. I don't think the other kids liked them either, some of the masks were made in the shape of Mickey Mouse but it didn't make me like them any better! We had to do our school work wearing them, it was very hard as the eye pieces kept misting up, and for me wearing glasses it was doubly difficult.

Dad was in THE HOME GUARD during the Second World War. I can see his rifle now standing in the corner of our sitting room, nobody would dream of touching it. We were warned of the consequences if we disobeyed this order. I used to love the warmth of Dad's Great-coat when it was used for a blanket on my bed on a cold winter night. I don't think for one moment it was supposed to be used in such a way, but I didn't care, all I knew was the big coat kept me toasty warm.

I remember the ration books and Mum swapping coupons with other mums, it was a regular thing back then. I didn't understand the full significance of what war meant, I did however realize what it was like to go to the sweet shop and find all the shelves empty. Sweets like lots of other things at the time were on ration. I remember mum buying the meagre ration of sweets, and putting the paper bag on the highest shelf in the larder, well out of the reach of little fingers.

I was a fat child, my hair was short and tied up in a ribbon, Mum wouldn't let me wear it long because of "nits (head lice)" ,she told me, which at that time were rife in the school. Scratching your head was all part and parcel of School life back then. I recall vividly every Friday night my brother and sister and I were subjected to a bath, a hair wash and our scalps scraped with the nit comb, kneeling over Mother's lap whilst she went nit picking onto a sheet of newspaper on her knee. This was to catch the little blighters. I will never forget the sound of nits being cracked between Mum's thumb-nails.

I wore glasses and I sported a pronounced squint, a classic combination for being bullied, and I was, on a regular basis. One of the favourite games for the bullies was to take my glasses from me, put them on the top of the outside school toilets, and make me sing to get them back. They frightened me a lot. I don't know what pleasure they derived from taunting me in this way; it was usually the older children who were the worst. I don't know how many times my glasses were either sprained by the tormenters twisting them or they had to be replaced because they had been broken by these cruel children!

To this day I feel sorry for any young child who has to wear glasses, and it crosses my mind as to whether they are tormented as I was although these days the glasses are in keeping with modern trends and can look like a fashion statement.

I will never forget one particularly hurtful incident to do with my glasses (mind you, this nasty bit of spite eventually brought about some welcome changes).

My glasses had been put in the usual out of place reach. At the same time these particular children had barred the way into the toilet and I wanted to wee. Teacher rang the bell to tell us to go to class. I got as far as the steps into the classroom and not being able to hold myself any longer I wet myself on the step! The woman teacher, having not one ounce of pity for me, made me wash my knickers in the toilet basin and hang them over the pipes to dry.

But the worst was to come. I was made to stand on a chair in front of the class. "Miss?" Then a wooden dummy was shoved in my mouth. This was a cruel sort of punishment, it was so big that it actually split my mouth at the sides. Some of the kids laughed some didn't. I remember to this day how worthless I was made to feel. Well, that was the start of better things for me.

My Mother fed up with me coming home crying, (I used to go home at play time almost every day at first, Mum having to take me back) went mad when I got home with a bleeding mouth. She marched into school the next morning rolled her cardigan sleeves up, and in front of teachers and kids or anyone else in the vicinity, smashed Miss Full in the Face! I suppose if she had done that these days she would have been in serious trouble. Mind you so would the school for allowing it!

After that things got better for me. I can't say I really enjoyed school at all. Arithmetic for me was a nightmare. I couldn't understand fractions, and even multiplying was a no-no. What I did quite like was writing. This was to stand me in good stead when many years later, in my sixties, I started writing in a serious way. Quite out of the blue, I managed to have some poetry published by a small company in America. Many years later I was to be published by two Christian publishers. Later I found a flare for writing children's stories.

Getting them published by CHIPMUNKA PUBLISHING gave me quite a buzz! I have Darin Jewell to thank for that. Darin was my agent for some time. It was he who put me in touch with CHIPMUNKA. Darin and I are still friends . We keep in contact. He helps me on occasion with a little problem that may come up from time to time. Looking back to my school days, it didn't matter that I could never get on with arithmetic. I was always able to look after my housekeeping money and I didn't need maths for writing and that's all that mattered to me!

P E was never my thing at School. For example I didn't like getting changed into the kit, and I could never master the vaulting horse, I usually got stuck on the top, due no doubt to me being plump. My Gran used to say to me when I asked her if I was fat, in her lovely way: "you're not fat love, you're just well covered". I adored my Granny, my sister, brother and I spent some lovely times at her house in Keighley where she lived with Granddad. Mum wasn't very well at times, she had two miscarriages besides losing baby Maureen, so I suppose, these were the times we spent holidays at

Granny's! I was to learn later, that Granny had looked after us at times when Mum was about other business!

I remember us being taken to Keighley by bus. I loved my time spent there. We always got off the bus in the town square, sometimes a market was being held. We got off the bus, and were soon caught up in the hustle and bustle. There were market stalls selling all sorts of wonderful things. There was a fruit stall selling bananas, we had never seen this fruit before. It must have been after the war, about 1946. The little man in a funny smock and hat was shouting out "a lovely bunch of bananas missus, 6 for a bob", that was about 5p in today's money. There was also an Italian man selling ice cream from a cart. He winked at me. I think that was the first time I had been winked at. I blushed in embarrassment. I was about 9 years old at the time. I remember Granny smiling at me as if she understood how I felt.

There were also some clothing stalls, and some selling handbags, and shoes. There was also a boy, trying to sell puppies. They were huddled in a cardboard box. I felt sorry for the poor little things. I would have loved one but Gran said they were probably sickly.

Granny's house was in Barry Street. To reach it we had to go down a long road from the town square. I remember the road sloped downwards between very high grey walls on either side. What fascinated me was the hollow sound of our shoes on the road as we made our way down. Eventually we reached a metal staircase, which took us up to Barry Street. It is really hard to explain, but the back of Granny's house could be seen high up as we made our way down the road. I never liked the climb up the twisted staircase

but once you reached the street up above it was fine. We were now on a different street level. The road was cobbled. To the left was the row of cottages where Granny lived. To the right a few streets sloped upwards towards another level. We used to go up there to play, the view from the very top was panoramic. You could see for miles to the rolling hills.

Granny and Granddad's house was very old and quite small. There were only two bedrooms, a sitting room, a scullery and a cellar. From the back scullery you could see right down to the road below.

Mum used to tell us the story of her having to clean the windows, when she was a girl. She had a fear of cleaning the ones in the scullery because she had to clean the outside whilst sitting on the window-sill and lean out while Granny held her legs. Looking down from that back window to the street far below, I can understand her fear! I wouldn't have wanted the job! At any price!

Two doors away from Granny's house at number three was where Granny's half sister lived, we used to call her Granny Walters. I didn't like her, she used to make her own cheese, the house stank of it. Granny used to send me for some of this foul smelling cheese because strangely enough my Granddad used to like it! I can see the place now. The kitchen table, with jugs of sour milk covered in muslin cloths as the stuff fermented into something resembling cream coloured sick! The smell permeated every corner of the small house. Granny Walters used to quiz me about my Granny, and what she was doing. I hated it. I don't think my Granny liked her half sister, she told me her Dad had married twice and Nellie, that was her half- sister's first name had always been jealous of her. She put up with her because Granddad liked the cheese she made. All I know is that every time I was asked to go to that stinking hovel I couldn't wait to get out.

Further down the street there was a lovely little woman by the name of Betty Carver. The thing that always used to fascinate my brother, sister and myself was the fact that her stomach almost touched the floor. She walked like a duck. When I asked my Granny why this was, she told me that the poor woman had had so many children. Three had died soon after birth, she had four left. Her stomach muscles had gone. Granny also said it was all down to Mr. Burt Carver, having an insatiable appetite for sex! Granny muttered something about "he would kill her one of these days." But I didn't really understand what that meant at the time.

Down at the bottom of Barry Street there was Bleach Factory. The chimney would regularly spew out the stench of strong chemicals. We used to hear the women who worked there going down the cobbled street in their wooden clogs. There was also The Knocker- upper, who tapped a long stick on bedroom windows to wake the sleeping girls in time for their shifts. I used to sleep in Granny and Granddad's bed. I had done from being a little girl. I remember at first the bed seemed so big with its flock mattress. Granddad used to lift me into the bed. Looking back, they couldn't have been very comfortable. I remember Granny telling

Granddad off for trumping in bed but I didn't care. I was at my Granny's, the best place on earth.

My Granddad used to study form, he would sit at the kitchen table, with piles and piles of newspapers, some had been there so long that they were yellow with age. To my knowledge he never won a penny on the horses. Granny used to ask him to get rid of some of the older ones but he was adamant. He would not hear of it. He would sit deep in thought, checking from this newspaper or one from another pile. Granddad had worked out many combinations of just which horse should win! However, as I said "he never won a Brass farthing!" as Granny was heard to say, to anyone who was interested enough to listen.

Another memory was of being sent to the shop on the corner across the road for gas mantles. There wasn't any electricity in the houses so people had candles and gas lamps. My Granny could never replace a mantle without putting her finger through the delicate structure. It used to fascinate me just how fragile the mantle was. Another lovely memory was when Granny used to make onion sandwiches for supper. She used to cut a big onion and soak the slices in a saucer full of vinegar. They were lovely.

It would turn out in later years after Granddad passed away that she would be coming to live with us for a while before she herself died of throat cancer.

Our school was called Greengate's Infants. It was up the hill from our house in Apperley Bridge. We lived in a rented, pebble dashed semi. Our house was in the centre of the row, it was a cul-de-sac so it was very safe to play in, with no through traffic. The only vehicles in our street were the Coal-man, the Baker and the occasional Shop on wheels which sold everything from paraffin to pots and pans, soap – powder and candles, in fact quite a bit of what you needed. I also remember the little man on his knife grinder at the end of our street. I used to watch the wheel going round, as it sharpened the knives, it made my teeth feel funny. I recall with nostalgia the horse-drawn milk-float with the old farmer wearing smock and gaiters, ladling milk from his churn into Mum's old jug. During the war years I only recall about two cars in our village. I remember with pleasure the times I played with my spinning top and coloured chalk. I loved to make new patterns and different shapes. Looking back at that time, some of the kids liked hopscotch, but it wasn't for me, I could play for a while but I used to lose my balance so it wasn't my favourite game. I quite liked playing with marbles, some of the colours were lovely, but there again I think this was a boy's game.

St John's Church was at one end of the village, and a Methodist Chapel at the other. My brother sister and I used to go to Chapel every Sunday morning. Dad sometimes took us to The Salvation Army on a Sunday evening. We had to catch a bus at the end of our street to go there. We had to go to Chapel whether we wanted to or not. Looking back on those long gone days it was probably the only time Mum had to herself.

I think the most tedious thing about Sunday, was having to put your best clothes on for Church in the morning, and take them off again at dinner time, only to repeat the action for the evening meeting at The Salvation Army Service, but I suppose that was what you did and that was all there was to be said.

There was the giant Cotton Mill just before you entered the village where I first started work at fourteen. There was also a Dry –Cleaner's factory by the side of the canal. My mum did a bit of cleaning there besides doing a bit at the pub. The railway station where my dad worked for a long time was situated across the road from the Chapel. There was a grocery shop where I used to buy single OXO CUBES. They were lovely to lick. Also we had a cake shop in our village where they sold the yummiest cream buns. We were allowed one for an occasional treat.

One day out of the blue, there was a massive fire at the Dry cleaning factory, a very traumatic time.

The factory, being only a stone's throw from our street, meant we were able to witness the whole thing.

It started at night. We were awakened by the commotion. Our bedroom wall felt warm to the touch. On looking out of our bedroom window we could see the factory full alight, and because it was on the banks of the canal the area directly in front was burning, due -I was informed later- to the chemicals from the factory seeping onto the canal. I had never seen water on fire before, it was frightening. Dad had got us all up, and we, along with other people of the village, most in their night attire, made our way to the fire. We were barred from going too close by the police and fire brigade.

I will never forget the man with his clothes on fire, jumping from the factory window into the burning canal. He must have died instantly because the canal was a mass of flames. The dryers and cleaners were destroyed. Lots of big tanks and other charred components belonging to the stricken factory were dumped in a field nearby.

Well us being kids, found these big tanks and other giant components made smashing playing material.
Dens and tunnels were constructed, mostly by the boys! So from total devastation for the factory workers, who had lost their jobs and in some cases their lives, it became absolute Heaven for us. We played daring games of Pirates, and other swashbuckling adventures on the make-believe ships, or castles with a drawbridge, so it fitted our childhood dreams.

We had a long back garden very useful for keeping chickens, ducks and bantams. We also had a noisy but tame cockerel. In fact a few of the chickens were quite tame. Lizzy, one of the largest hens used to come into the kitchen. She also liked to watch for worms as Dad dug in the garden.

One fateful day my sister at about the age of five was helping Dad, and asked if she could do some digging. Dad handed her the spade, telling her to be careful. Lizzy was standing close by as she always did... Sandra, not looking what she was doing stuck the spade into the soil, there arose an enormous squawk from the startled hen as my sister cut off one of her claws! Well Lizzy did recover but from then on she stayed well away from the spade, especially when Sandra was helping! A little earlier when my sister was about three, she did something that turned my stomach. Dad used to catch slugs and snails in the garden and put them on the path, put salt on their tails to kill them. Sandra picked up a juicy snail and ate it, slime running from her mouth. Mum went mad, trying to wash my sister's mouth out, but Sandra didn't seem to suffer any ill effects.

Another trying time for one of the hens happened when she got something stuck in her throat, almost costing her her life, had it not been for Dad's quick action on that day that is what would have happened!
He took hold of the choking bird and slit an opening in her craw. He took out the offending piece of food, and with a needle and white cotton sewed the cut up! Amazingly the hen lived quite happily for a number of

years after that, I don't know how Dad would have got on today. He would probably be up before the law for animal cruelty! He was a bit of an idiot and had a wonderful sense of humour. Sometimes his jokes left Mum cold, but we kids used to laugh at him.

Winters were very cold and it was not unusual to have lots of heavy snow. During the winter of 1947 snow had fallen for days, my most vivid recollection is of my dad and other dads having to dig paths between the houses. Snow was as high as a grown man. Of course for we kids it was magic, trying to walk through the maze of tunnels created by the hard packed snow. I also remember with a smile the sledges Dad made for us out of bits of wood, the best one being the one with an old drawer nailed to a base.

Our village was surrounded by hills, ideal for sledging down. We also had a lot of dry stone walls. I dragged my sledge to the top of a hill with quite a gradient, five in one I think (well that's what I heard people say). I set off picking up speed as I careered downwards. I hit one of the dry stone walls at the bottom head on. It was completely covered in deep snow. All I remember after that was a loud bang and me sailing over the top of the hidden wall on the now loose drawer. I suffered a few bruises but that was all.

One lovely memory was Dad taking me mushroom picking, we used to go ever so early in the morning, Dad said it was the best time to go. I loved the taste of bacon, eggs and mushroom, and looking back he knew instinctively, which of these mushrooms were poisonous, and which were safe to eat. He never picked a wrong one! I used to think my dad was clever, in more ways than one!

Another momentous occasion to come to mind was when our landlord wanted someone to paint the windows and doors of the houses in our street. There were twenty five houses in all including a sweet shop at the end of the street, this was owned by a family who gave the impression of being a cut above every body else in our street. They were the first family to have a television. All us kids used to stand on their garden wall looking into their front room hoping to catch a glimpse of this wonderful innovation. We got sent off on many occasions.

Dad was a dab hand at most things, so he volunteered his services for the job. He was supplied with lots of tins of what he said were battleship blue in colour. I can see him now as he climbed ladders to the upper floors of every property in the street. I remember him being tired and complaining of aches and pains and sporting a few blisters on his hands, but he completed the task in a decent time. Dad said with the money he received for doing the job, he could take us to Scarborough to Uncle Harry and Aunty Nellie's Boarding House for a couple of weeks in the School holidays.

We went to Scarborough quite a few times during our childhood. I really enjoyed it. One particular holiday at my Uncle's a few Americans were staying there. One day whilst they were talking to Uncle Harry, one of them gave Mum a tin of fudge. I remember the tin being opened at each end and the roll of delicious fudge pushed through onto a tea plate. We kids loved this sweet unusual treat, it was cut into slices like cake, it was lovely. I used to like to hear the Americans speaking as well, quite different from our broad Yorkshire accent.

On a particularly hard Winter's day it was quite usual to have thick ice inside as well as on the outside windows. I used to breathe on my fingers and try to rub a hole on the ice that had formed overnight on the bedroom window pane, in order to look out. I didn't have much success though as it was even colder on the other side of the glass, so the ice was thicker.   Winters were much colder in Yorkshire back then.

We didn't have central heating in those days. What we did have though was a lovely fire in our front room.

Dad also used to mend our shoes with pieces of thick rubber on his LAST, this was a type of contraption used by cobblers. I think the pieces of rubber came from old car tires but I can't be certain. He used to smoke like a chimney. He would sometimes send me to the shop with two pence halfpenny, for five Woodbines (in old money).   Mum used to tell him off for leaving his fags burning in the house, every window-sill was covered in fag burns and ash . No wonder we all had bronchitis!

I watch with nostalgia now, episodes of DAD'S ARMY on television.   Some of the antics of this lovable lot of clowns are so reminiscent of the things my dad used to get up to. We used to watch this intrepid bunch of soldiers, marching down the road in the middle of our village, as they practiced this maneuver or another marching drill. I was so proud of my dad, but couldn't help laughing at the different shapes and sizes of the men. Old Harry Bancroft was as long and as thin as a twig, while Mr. Andrews was as fat as pudding. There was a lot of talk about THE BLACK MARKET and Mr. Charlie Andrews being involved, but I didn't know what it meant.

When the war finally came to an end there was much rejoicing with street parties and bonfires. The road to victory had been a long and hard one but after almost six years of global conflict the allies prevailed.

The war came to an end in Europe on the 8th May 1945. There was much rejoicing on the home front.

Millions of Britons had endured much hardship. They had dug and planted, grown their own vegetables, gone without many things. Blackout curtains were taken down from windows and doors.

It was decided by the men of the village that they would build a big bonfire in our street to celebrate the end of the war, so wood was collected for the grand fire. Dad provided old sleepers from the railway where he worked, as a signalman. I can still visualize what happened next. Dad placed a large piece of wood containing big nails sticking out of it up against our garden wall. Using a large chopper he began to chop it. Well you can guess what happened next, with a mighty swipe he hit the piece of wood, the top piece containing most of the rusty nails, sailed into the air and came down cutting Dad's left ear away from his face. I screamed in terror, I was convinced that Dad had lost his ear for good, I felt sick!

Dad yelled out in agony, and I suppose fear, he was cupping his cut ear in his hand, and the blood dripped freely down. He was taken to hospital by one of the dads who owned a car. His ear was stitched back on. When the evening came round and the festivities began Dad swathed in bandages tried to laugh it off. I will never forget the blood and Mum's worried face and angry voice as she chastised him for being so stupid.

The fire was lit, along with the fireworks. It was a smashing party, that was until the flames shot up into the night sky. The fire had got a lot bigger than expected, nobody noticed that the newly painted houses were beginning to blister . Potatoes that had been thrown into the fire were raked out and judging by the black mouths of the kids, they had been eaten with glee, even though they were only partly cooked!

The following day the landlord was not very pleased and Dad had to paint some of the houses again.

Mum reckoned that had the landlord not felt sorry for Dad then he would have had to pay for the replacement paint with his own money! It wasn't funny at the time but the incident has caused much laughter to people over the years. After a time Dad's ear healed and you couldn't see a scar.

Another trying time for me was when I was about ten years old. I had been ill with a sore throat for some time, it got much worse and I remember Dad putting my bed downstairs. I suppose it was easier for Mum to look after me. The doctor came to see me a few times. I was getting worse. Dad came home from work at the railway station. He put his head round the door and looked at me. I remember vividly telling him I was dying.

Mum had put a bucket or a bowl down earlier because I was feeling sick. I could hardly swallow or breathe for the awful pain in my throat! I had a strange sensation of being above myself, looking down, it was a warm safe, out of pain feeling.

All of a sudden I was back in my bed and coughed up a lot of blood. I was covered in it. I was also very frightened. From then on I began to get better. I had recovered from Diphtheria. This was a known killer at the time. I remember my granny telling me it hadn't been my time. God didn't want me just yet!

It took a long time for me to recover to full health but I suppose I was fortunate for at that time in the 1940s Diphtheria was a known killer.

We used to have big celebrations for MAY DAY back then, we used to dress up in fancy dress, and receive prizes for the best out-fit. Our bicycles were trimmed up with coloured crepe paper. Girls who had dolls' prams also had them dressed in this fancy paper. We had sports day on the same day. I never cared for that because I wasn't very sporty, not built for it. I hated wearing shorts, my legs not being my best feature.

Some of the men did walking races, this from the back looked hilarious, their different sized bottoms waggling up and down as they passed you by, their elbows sticking out at the side, it was comical...

Another incident was hilarious in content and has been remembered and laughed about by my brother, sister and I ever since it happened. Now after all these years we still feel the memory sweet in the telling. We were coming home from school one afternoon. There were about six of us altogether, we were all going in the same direction because we were close neighbours.

The road from the school sloped down quite sharply into the village. As we strolled home, not rushing but playing about as kids do, there was a farmer's field. Now because of the steepness of the road cutting down beneath the field, we were unable to see the cow standing right above us by the side of the field. We had stopped and were mucking about. What we failed to notice was the cow's bum perched over the side of the wall. It was now directly above us. One of the younger boys was wearing a knitted balaclava helmet, and was unfortunately in the firing line.

Without warning there was a loud splosh, as the cow relieved herself of the steaming poo all over young Barry Hargrieves! Well unfortunately because of the volume of cow manure, the balaclava hat he was wearing had little effect in protecting the poor lad. He was covered from head to foot in smelly runny dung! I will never forget his face as he tried to open his eyes and mouth.

Kids can be cruel and despite his cries nobody would take him home, because none of us wanted to be anywhere near that stink!

Somebody did go and fetch his mum though, and he was taken home, stripped of the smelly clothes, and put into the tin bath in the yard... His mother must have had a hard job cleaning the lad up. As to his poo stained clothes I never did find out how the poor woman managed to get them clean! You couldn't afford to throw clothes away in those days.

Mum was rather strict in some ways, and I have to smile when I think of yet another incident that would make my brother sit up. He was about seven at the time, I was nine. We were at the Saturday Morning Picture House. We called it the "Flee-pit" for reasons that don't need any explaining! Brian was sitting with his friend. I was with a girl across the isle just one or two rows behind him. He and the other boy were smoking cigarettes and puffing away for all they were worth. Brian was sitting back in his seat with his legs pressed against the seat in front of him.

The curtain had just gone up and the introductory music was playing loudly. We were getting ready to watch the next exciting episode of ROY ROGERS AND TRIGGER. The next thing I saw was mum rushing past me, grabbing hold of my brother, and lifting him over the back of his seat. Brian was so shocked, he hadn't expected that. I can see and hear Mum to this day:

"I WILL TEACH YOU NOT TO SMOKE FILTHY CIGARRETTES MY LAD" she said. This message went with a clip round the ear with every word. I never saw my brother with a fag after that.

Another time worth a mention, if only to tell others what happens when you don't do as your dad tells you. I was about nine. Dad had been mending the front wheel of my bike. Dad said not to use the bike again until he had mended it. Well I was going to chapel, which was situated at the top of the hill. I wanted my bike. So when dad wasn't looking I sneaked off. I always pushed the bike up the hill because it was very steep. It was ok going up so I couldn't see why Dad had been so adamant about not taking it.

I was to find out why in a very hard and painful way. I came out of chapel after the service. My bike was leaning up against the chapel wall where I had left it. I wheeled it to the edge of the road, got on it sat on the saddle and set off. I hadn't gone many feet, when to my horror the front wheel went running down the hill on its own. The frame that had been holding it smashed with a screaming thud onto the road. The next thing, I flew over the handle-bars landing on my face onto the road, breaking my glasses, and badly cutting my face arms and legs. Two or three boys passed me but ignored my cries for help. Seconds later, a bus came up the hill and ran over what was left of my bike. This had happened out side the pub where Dad worked part time. The Inn keeper and his wife saw what had happened. They came out to me, picked me up, and they took me and, what was left of my bike, home. Mum called the doctor, who dressed my wounds, and said he would be back in a few days, meanwhile I was to stay in bed. Well it turned out that I stayed in bed for almost two weeks, my eyes black and my body bruised and hurting, and after that I had to visit the doctors and the eye specialist. I had to have new glasses aswell! I learned later that the bus driver had stopped and given all the relevant information to the police.

What I wasn't aware of until my sister Sandra enlightened me recently was that she and my Brother Brian had been standing by the pub at the time! She tells me that I came flying down the steep hill at about 100 miles an hour. She said it looked hilarious, that was until the front tyre went careering down the road, and I went flying over the handlebars, landing on my face! She said she remembers the gravel being picked out of my face and leg.

I left school at fourteen without any qualifications at all, but that didn't matter to me, I was going to work in the Cotton Mill just up the road from our house. I didn't need a degree in anything for that job.

The hours were 8am until 6 pm, the wage was meagre for the hours worked. After giving Mum my pay packet I ended up with about 9 shillings (45p in today' s money) but it was still enough to buy my stockings or a magazine or some other bits and bobs a young girl of the time needed.

The work was noisy, dirty and hard. To me the giant looms looked enormous. My job was to pull the bobbin away from the thick leather belt that went round the machines at a terrific speed. Then as quickly as I could

I had to thread the cotton through the Doffers and Twisters. These were the components that sent the cotton to the big reels above. Because of my age I had to go to the rest room for a little while every few hours. Jim the foreman was a stickler for this rule. He said it was to give me a rest because of the noise.

Whilst working there I got an infection just by my elbow. I had a scab as big as a teacup for quite a long time.

Another upsetting time for me is worth a mention before I go any further.

I had also started my "monthlies" early (whilst I was still at school.) This was the term used in those days for monthly periods. Mine started when I was 11 years old. One school morning, when I was at the local baths, for swimming lessons I remember taking my clothes off to put my costume on. There was blood in my knickers and I thought I was dying. My mum hadn't said anything to me about this perfectly natural occurrence. You didn't talk about such things back then.   My only sex education from my mum was, and not until the bleeding:

 "get this piece of rag on, put it in your pants, wash it out when it's dirty and put it over the washing line".

 I remember the pieces of rag neatly folded for comfort. I think mum made them from warn sheets. It wasn't a very nice job washing the bits of cloth, but I suppose it was cheaper than buying sanitary towels from the shop. I also recall her stern warning "Keep away from the boys, this will happen every month or so from now ". It became a bit of a bind when working in the filthy conditions of the mill trying to change these bits of rag when I had a period, and wrap the dirty ones up to take home to wash. When I started to earn my own money, I was able to buy my own and stop the horrible job of washing bloody smelly rags. It was a relief to be able to buy shop ones, disposing the soiled ones down the toilet pan.! It was quite an innovation to wear a sanitary belt. Very modern! What wasn't very clever on my part though was once I thought it would be a good idea to put neat DETTOL onto my sanitary towel, it would be a way of stopping any other smell. Well I can tell you it wasn't the best idea I ever had, within a few minutes of putting it on, I was aware of a burning stinging feeling in my knickers. I was soon at the kitchen sink washing myself below with warm water and Mum's green soap. That was the last time I tried that daft trick. I was about twelve at the time. But you live and learn don't you!

Well I can tell you I was horrified at the thought of this bleeding every month. I didn't care much for the nagging tummy ache either. Why did I have to keep away from the boys? They didn't bother me anyway. They never had except to make fun of me. There was one boy I had played with ever since I was a little girl, he was the only one who didn't call me 'fatty four eyes', or some other nasty name, despite the fact that earlier my brother had given him a pair of my navy blue knickers to go swimming in! This had caused a titter with the kids, apparently they had said amongst themselves that they could all fit into them at the same time! This is another gem my sister enlightened me with recently! Thankfully we have all been blessed with a sense of humour, it comes from Dad.

I liked Billy, he was great we used to play on the old barge down on the canal sometimes with a couple of other kids, but this little adventure didn't last very long, we were snitched on by some of the village boys. This particular afternoon, we were sat on the broken and gradually submerging barge, when in the distance I saw my mum and Billy's aunty Beth coming along the tow path, followed by the kids who'd told on us.

As my mum came closer I saw her face, it was white with anger. I felt sick. Billy and I walked gingerly across the slim bridge that went from one side of the lock to the path at the other side. My mum grabbed hold of me, in front of all the kids who had followed behind hoping no doubt we would both receive a good hiding. They weren't disappointed! My mum did no more than bend me down, pull my navy knickers up over the left cheek of my bum and give me a few hard smacks, much to the delight of the snotty nosed kids

who were looking on! Billy got a few cuffs round his head from Aunty Beth. For ages after that embarrassing episode, the village kids would taunt me with , "we've seen Dot's fat arse."

Sometimes we would go bird nesting with other kids from the village, but I didn't like that much, it was taking the baby chicks away that wasn't nice. I always felt sorry for the mother birds, but back then it was quite acceptable to go bird nesting! I remember my brother Brian showing me how to pierce a hole in both ends of the egg and blow out the contents. Trouble was if you sucked instead of blew the contents of the egg, the taste in your mouth wasn't very nice.

Billy lived with his dad and Aunty Beth, down the lane from us. We weren't supposed to be on the old barge it was dangerous. I had been warned many times. Besides for some reason, not understood by me at the time, I was warned never to play with this particular boy. He came from a bad family. Of course I came to realize later, that his dad and aunty were as they used to say in those days, "living over the brush" (not married) but I was unaware of such things and the implications back then. It was a different kind of life to the one we live these days. Was it better back then? In some ways I think it probably was!

As we reached our teens thing and feelings began to change. Billy was about sixteen and I was fifteen, we had played together for years, getting up to all sorts of things, pinching apples from Old Grady's orchard, if he caught you he would box your ears. However, this particular Sunday Billy asked me to go for a walk in the woods. He would meet me from chapel. Well this was ok, so I said yes. Billy was waiting outside for me. He was dressed in his best clothes. I felt funny. I wasn't used to seeing Billy dressed in anything but his old stuff, or school uniform. As we approached Bluebell wood Billy got hold of my hand. He leaned towards me and tried to kiss me. That was it! The childhood friendship had taken on an embarrassing change. I didn't like it. This was a much different Billy from the one I had always felt at ease with!

From then on everything was changed. I couldn't be with Billy anymore! I suppose in grownup terms I didn't fancy him in that way, whatever that way was. I had never thought of Billy in any other way than as my friend! Nothing had ever crossed my mind in a sexual nature to do with him. Billy had a bit of a bad reputation, but I didn't care, he had been my friend until the walk in the woods had changed everything!

I knew nothing back then about life and hurting love. I was to find out these things later on in my own life. In the years to come I would suffer hurting devastating love that almost sent me crazy. I fought with God for him, but lost the battle, I also battled with the devil and his tormenting wiles. I eventually won a sort of peace I was able to live with. Thankfully up to then, I was unaware of what was to come.

One day my sister, brother and I were all playing in the field across the road from our house. In the corner of the field there was a pig sty. One of the boys removed the pixy hat my sister was wearing and threw it into the sty. My brother took his brother's school cap and chucked that in amongst the pigs. Well eventually all hell was let loose and about ten kids ended up being thrown in to the slime. By the time my mum and a few other mums arrived on the scene, the place was bedlam. Kids covered in pig muck and mud were all fighting amongst the frightened pigs.

Well I can tell you! My brother and sister and I were all put in the bath. We all had a smacked bum and got sent to bed. It must have been some job for Mum to get us, and our soiled clothes clean and smelling fresh again.

My Dad had worked as a signalman at the local railway for a good many years.

One of my special memories of that time was taking my dads' snack to the signal-box .The railway station was only just up the road from our house so the journey was a short one. I can still recall, after all these years, the thrill of seeing the smoke belching from the funnel as the mighty train passed under the signal-box. There was a special smell to the inside of the small interior, perhaps it was the oily rag Dad used to grab hold of the levers, as he maneuvered the tracks into place. I always told him he had the arms of Popeye, the famous cartoon character of the time. However, I never did get used to the mighty leviathans steaming their thunder into the station. If I happened to be on the platform with my dad as the monster came screaming down the track in front of us, I would stand behind him for protection.

He also worked part time at the local village pub as a barman. I remember how smart he looked in his black suit. The jacket had tails as I remember and he also wore a white shirt with a 'Dicky-bow tie.' He always put a neatly folded white handkerchief in his top pocket and his shoes were always highly polished.

Mum also worked part time doing a bit of cleaning or sometimes in the evening if there was a special party at the pub, she would put on her best frock and help behind the bar. Aunty Ivy would always look after my younger sister, brother and I on these special evenings.

I suppose the extra money came in very useful. Mum was a good cook so we regularly had homemade rabbit stew and veg. It was fine when I was a child but the thought of eating rabbit turned my stomach later, when that horrible disease to cut down the rabbit population was introduced by a very cruel regime. Years later, when riding in our car in the country and seeing a poor rabbit in the middle of the road with bulging eyes, going round in a circle looking very tragic my hubby didn't stop the car and we felt the bump as the wheels went over the poor thing. Joe, my then husband said it was the kindest thing to do. I wept for quite a time for the hapless creature.

Sometimes we enjoyed a chicken from our back garden, nearly every one had chickens and ducks. It was nothing to hear the raucous rattle of a cockerel coming from a garden nearby. He would wake us up regularly early in the morning but that was ok, it was all part of life back then.

I remember us kids having to clean out our own chicken pen, a horrible smelly job, but we had to do it like it or not. Brian always did his best to get out of the stinking job.

We had a scrubbed wooden table in our kitchen; it was used for a variety of jobs. On baking day it was used to rollout the pastry, on ironing day it was used, covered in a thick cloth, to smooth out the clothes and sheets, with the old electric iron plugged into the light above the table. Using an extension, it was possible to have the light on too, quite modern, for those times.

The old table was used for a much more gruesome job, this one upset us kids quite a bit. We weren't supposed to witness it but I came in from play one day to see Dad chop the head off one of the chickens. When he could see how upset it made me, he tried to make me feel better by telling me it wasn't one of our own birds. The worst thing about it was, when the head had been severed the chicken ran headless round the table before it collapsed... Dad said it was the nerves that made the bird run and it could no longer feel anything. I have never been convinced of this fact! Mind you, I wasn't averse to playing with the claws that had been cut off the poor chicken, if you pulled the tendon, the claws moved in and out. I have never forgotten that episode.

Another thing worth a mention, one day we had a fuse go in the box in the kitchen. Dad, without any thought for his welfare, climbed the ladder he had brought in from the tool shed and stuck the blade of a kitchen knife into the electric box. The next thing to happen was that he yelled out in agony, fell from the ladder , onto the floor, and I remember the smell of burnt flesh . Dad had a burn in the middle of his hand from the steel knife. My dad was an idiot. Mum went mad and called him all the names she could lay her tongue to!

Another job for us was picking red and white currants for Mrs. Wilder who lived next door. I didn't like this tedious job. The only reason for helping was the promise of a bag of fried new potatoes each. The conical bags were just the job, you could drink the vinegar that had collected in the point of the bag.

Mrs Wilder cooked them herself in her chip pan. Lovely!

When I was about eleven. Dad decided he had had enough of the railway and the part time job in the village pub. He applied for a job in a posh Hotel in South Harrow. I used to hear Mum and Dad arguing in their bedroom, I once saw mum throw a dinner plate right across the kitchen at Dad. He ducked, and the plate smashed against the opposite wall. I suppose she didn't want him to go, that was what the rows were about.

Anyway he did get his way and he did go to this new job. I missed him so much. I suppose we all did. Gran used to come and stay quite regularly, this was smashing. Granny was lovely. I have a memory of Mum feeling faint one day and Granny pushing her head down onto her lap. I also remember Granny telling Mum to pull herself together, for the sake of the kids! It's only when you grow up, that you realize just what it must have been like for Mum to bring us three up on her own.

The war hadn't been over very long, so things must have been tight. Rationing was still on for some things... Bread that hadn't been rationed during the war was put on ration for two years in 1946. This was due to the fact that there was a worldwide grain shortage.

In the second half of the 1940s things were as bad as they had been in the war; long queues were in fact a part of everyday life. They used to say: "see a queue and join it " so people did, you never knew what you just might find , it could be anything that was in short supply.

Another thing Mum made us kids do, which we didn't particularly enjoy, was to take the old pram and a shovel and go to the yard of the metal-box factory and fetch slack and tiny bits of coal from the huge pile that was used to keep the factory fires going. I don't suppose for one minute we were entitled to steal it, but we weren't the only ones who turned up with a pram. If they were aware of the goings on at the factory, I never knew. All I remember was that the pile of slack never seemed to be any less! And we always had a warm fire in the winter.

So this is what Mum was left with, and she resented the fact that Dad was away from it all.   I think Dad had wanted a change of scene, but it was hard for Mum. Dad did send money home on a regular basis, he came home every few months. He even sent us clothes and little presents. Once he sent me a lovely pair of blue and white summer shoes. Very smart! I went out to play in them much against Mum's orders. We were by the canal. My brother said: "let's see if your shoes will float", I didn't think it was a good idea, but went along with it anyway. Brian put my lovely shoes in the water, and they sank like stones!   We both had a good hiding for that little prank. I never saw my shoes again. And I had only worn them once!   No wonder Mum was angry.

As time went on, months into years, it was obvious that Mum was getting more and more fed up. It wasn't until I grew up myself and had children of my own, that the true significance of bringing children up really hit me. It must have been very hard for Mum coping on her own. Granny came to stay a lot, but all the same being without Dad finally got to Mum so one day, out of the blue, we were informed that our furniture was being put into storage and we were going to live in South Harrow. The shock to us kids was traumatic. All we had known was our sleepy village, and our lives there. We were going somewhere strange, it wouldn't be our lovely village anymore, and it was scary.   To this day I will never forget my granny waving us off from the train station. It would be a long time before we saw her again.

CHAPTER 2

THE START OF CHANGE

The train arrived at VICTORIA STATION. The journey had been exciting but I think I was still in shock. This was a foreign place to us. I remember walking in front of Mum along the noisy platform. I was sixteen years old at the time, Brian was fourteen and Sandra was eleven. I had left the cotton mill. Probably it was the best thing. If I had stayed in Yorkshire it would more than likely have been my lifetime's work for as I mentioned before, most of the older women who had worked in the mill for years were as deaf as posts. That would have no doubt been my fate.

Dad came out of smoke and the people milling around the platform. He put his arms around me. I noticed Mum hanging back. Brian and Sandra rushed to Dad's side. We had all missed him terribly. His words to me gave me a shock

"I don't know what your mother thinks she's playing at?" I remember feeling awkward. What did he mean? I don't think my brother and sister heard what he said. They were just happy to see Dad. He went towards

Mum took the case she was carrying and said something but he didn't kiss her. I was beginning to feel a bit scared, this wasn't right.

We walked from the station and Dad called a taxi. We all jumped in. Mum still looking tight faced.

After a while we arrived at our destination. Dad had left the posh pub some time earlier, in favour of being the boss of his own social club. Well that's what we thought! It would come to light at a later time, that Dad had been up to no good with a woman who owned the posh pub. Apparently a well wisher had informed Mum of this fact earlier on with a letter she had sent to her back home! Hence the move, and Mum's tight face! We all got out of the taxi. We were standing in front of a nondescript building with the sign over the club entrance flashing on and off.

Dad paid the taxi fare and ushered us all inside the front door. We stood in a lobby and looked around. To me it didn't seem up to much. Dad opened another door to the side of the lobby. We were shown inside this grotty room. It wasn't very big; there were three beds and a bit more furniture. There was green lino on the floor and there was one small window. What sent alarm bells ringing was that on the windows were steel bars! When I asked Dad what they were for, he said, "safety love, it's a bit of a rough area."   Well it turned out that Dad had been ill prepared for Mum's determination to make him stand up to his responsibilities. She had decided that enough was enough.   Especially after the letter informing Mum about Dad's little dalliance!

Later on in life I realized that life isn't black and white there are many shades, in fact, it's just life!
There was no room for Brian or Dad in the small room I was sleeping in with Sandra and Mum, so they slept under the pool table by the side of the dance floor. Brian has mentioned to me lately that he hated the way we were living, and that he had really missed our home in Yorkshire.   It has to be said though the kitchen had all the modern conveniences so I suppose that was a bonus.

Dad trying to make the best of things asked a question there really was no answer to.   Looking at us kids, he said, "do you think you can make this your new home?" I felt sick, how could this place be home when we had left behind our lovely home in Yorkshire?   I hated it, there was a feeling of something not very nice and an undercurrent of something going on!   Well of course there was, but we kids didn't know quite what at the time!

After we had been living in this nightmare way, I woke up one morning in this horrible damp room to find I was unable to straighten my legs. I was in excruciating pain and my fingers resembled sausages. The doctor was called and I was rushed into EDGEWARE GENERAL HOSPITAL where I stayed for about four months. Rheumatic fever was diagnosed. I was told when I had been there for three and a half months that if this certain test came back ok I could go home in two weeks. That was the start of my nervous problems. I was frightened that if the test was negative, I wouldn't be able to leave the hospital. My stay in hospital had been traumatic.

It wasn't long after that episode Dad found us some rooms but it was obvious after a time that the people we were lodging with were getting fed up. My brother and dad stayed on sleeping in the club so it was only Mum my sister and myself. I could tell that we weren't wanted there. There was always an undercurrent of bad feeling, probably because they were aware of Dad's affair with this married woman!

The most sickening thing for me at that time was when Mum gave me a letter to read she had found in Dad's coat pocket. With the words" there Dorothy, that's your precious father for you," it spoke of sexual things that were going to happen next time he met this woman.

I didn't really understand at the time, but instead of it turning me against my dad, it was my mother I hated for showing me this letter.   Mum actually cut her wrists, with a kitchen knife, it wasn't bad and it didn't bleed much, I think it was a token of how hopeless Mum felt, I remember putting a bandage on both wrists and actually at one point having to slap her face because she became hysterical.

It was only years later when I had experienced what hurting passion can do, that I am able to
understand what it must have been like for Mum and Dad during that upsetting time. I don't think my brother and sister will remember much if anything about this time in our lives. Well I hope they don't anyway. I love them both very much. When we occasionally get together the talk turns to our childhood and the things we used to get up to. We usually laugh until we cry.

We stayed in South Harrow until January 1954. We were all relieved to be leaving that horrible place with all its bad memories well and truly behind us. I know from what my brother has told me only recently, that he was very unhappy in that place, so when Dad got another position in another town we were all relieved.

The only good thing to come out of that place in South Harrow was an abandoned collie-cross puppy. She seemed to take to us so we brought her with us, she was about five months old and all black with the kindest eyes.

Dad had wisely decided on a change of job and location. I think he was fed up with the hassle. He realized that he had mucked up big time and things had to change. He had applied for and got a job for them both: steward and stewardess of a WORKING MEN'S CLUB in a place on the outskirts of The Cotswolds. On a cold February morning we set off. We didn't have a car, Dad couldn't drive anyway so we all climbed into the removal van. I will never forget the relief at finally leaving that horrible place behind.

As we travelled, snow was falling fast. Brian wanted to wee rather badly so Mum told him to use an empty pop bottle. After about two hours the driver stopped so we could have a good stretch. Mum without much ado, emptied the wee onto the snow. That was the first time I had seen yellow snow. The driver had pulled up in a lay by. We all jumped out the dog included. The snow was quite thick , the dog seemed very interested in a particular patch of snow. She began to dig furiously. What she found, was to give the dog her name. Mum went to see what was so interesting only to find about four or five wet bank notes where the dog had been digging. That is how she got the name Lucky. We dried the notes out and mum found good use for them, including a treat for all of us and a bone for Lucky.

We arrived at our destination mid afternoon. It was still snowing. We piled out of the van and into our new home. The van driver and his mate soon had the van unloaded, placing our furniture in the rooms that Mum pointed out. It was almost like home again. The three-piece suite and the sitting room carpet almost fitted our new room. It was nice to see familiar things around us once more.

We were in a lovely little market town, old world buildings steeped in history, were all around us. Back then in the 1950s the town was truly alive with hustle and bustle with a character all of its own. I remember lying in my bed on that first morning listening to local fishermen as they gathered on the wall below me. We lived quite close to the river, so I think the club was a meeting place to set off from and return to, after a day's fishing.   The Working Men's Club back in those days was quite olde worlde, the bar room, retaining its charm, with the old stone floor, and old-fashioned décor.

One memory that stays with me, is one that Mum, never managed to live down. The customers at the time, have mostly passed on now. They used to pass bags of produce over the bar to Mum, potatoes, spring onions and the like.   One day not long after we had moved in, one of the old boys passed a carrier of asparagus over the bar.   We had never seen this vegetable before. Mum cooked some for our dinner the following day. None of us liked it, we found it tough and bitter, it was much later that Mum found she had thrown the wrong end away. She was the butt of a few jokes after that! In fact I don't think she ever really lived it down.

We hadn't been in Evesham very long, about eighteen months, when my Granny came to live with us.

Earlier that year we had all suffered a death in the family. An uncle and aunty had spent time with us when they had come from Yorkshire on Uncle's motorbike. Granny had lived with them since Granddad had passed away. As they got about eight miles from home on their return journey, the vehicle got onto a patch of oil. My aunty fell off the back of the bike and died instantly. When Uncle got back to Granny and told her what had happened the shock was so great, it was believed that this was the start of her cancer, she had been a big lady about seventeen stone. As I have already stated Uncle George didn't last very long without Olive. No way would Granny be able to cope on her own so she came to stay with us.

When this feeble old lady walked into our porch at the club we could hardly believe it was the same woman. Granny was gaunt and looked really ill. Her clothes were dropping off her. I put my arms round this stick like woman and cried.

I have sad memories of my Granny not being able to eat solid food; she had to be fed through a tube into her stomach. I will never forget feeding her with a liquid supplement through this tube. It was poured into the top via a funnel and squeezed down with a sort of softball, attached to the tube. I can see the look of hopelessness on her face now, as one of us was feeding her, usually Mum or I and the thought still has the power to upset me, even after all these years. I particularly remember the piece of sticking plaster that held the tube to the top of her chest. The piece of tubing was permanently in her stomach, through a hole in her side, barbaric by today's standards, but this was well over fifty years ago. Gran had been a strong lady so it must have been very hard for her. Mind you I am not surprised she had this illness, I remember her rolling her own cigarettes. She used to ask anybody for their tab ends to put in her roller, in those days most working class people smoked so friends and family would oblige. I can see her now with her green fag papers making her roll ups. She had a tin box for all her fag ends. It used to fascinate me, her skill with the roller and paper was never to be forgotten.

My brother and sister being younger than me seemed to take the move from Yorkshire to South Harrow, then to Evesham in their stride. I don't know if they found the change of location upsetting. Perhaps it was more of an adventure for them but whereas I had to find work, they went to the local school just over the road from THE CLUB. Brian has mentioned to me lately how much he had hated being in that awful club sleeping under the pool table, and also at the school in Harrow. Kids were cruel to him because of his Northern accent but I think my brother and sister settled well at the school in our new permanent home in Evesham. They were glad no doubt to have left that horrible place in South Harrow far behind them.

Back home in Yorkshire I had been working in a cotton mill from the age of fourteen. The camaraderie had been great in the Mill back in my lovely village. Mind you, having said that, I don't think I would have wanted to make the Mill my life's work. Most of the people, who had worked there for years, were as deaf as a post and talked with hand signs. This used to fascinate me when I first started work there. It was strange to see women who were waving franticly to each other over the machinery. They had impaired hearing due to the constant noise of the looms.

I had worked there for almost two years and because of my age and the sheer hard work I had to have longer rests than the older women. The foreman Jim made sure that I took the rests. He said to me "it's the law girl, and we must abide by the law". Jim was a stickler for the rules. Some of the old women were a bit catty and resented my time in the rest room. I can't say I blamed them, they could probably have done with more rest time themselves!

The first job of work I found in Evesham was in a little haberdashery shop but I didn't really like it. The other two shop assistants in the boutique were older than me and 'talked posh', and to be honest I don't think my broad Yorkshire twang went down very well with these girls who had lived in Evesham all their lives. I was accused of talking to the customers too much and I was asked to leave by the manager, not very nice, when you are only sixteen. I remember my Mum storming into the shop and telling the stuck up manager his fortune, but it was to be the best thing that could have happened to me at the time.

After that I got a job in a needle factory about fifteen miles away in Redditch. I had to travel every day in the back of a van with three men, I didn't like the job or the mode of traveling and packed it in.

Then I managed to get a cleaning job in the local cottage hospital where I stayed for quite a while
 (this lovely old building was raised to the ground many years ago in favour of housing.)

I loved this work. I could chat to the patients inbetween mopping floors and washing walls and lockers. In those days good old-fashioned bleach did a wonderful job of keeping things clean. We never heard of super bugs in those days. Everything was kept absolutely pristine. The old fashioned Matron, was a force to be reckoned with but my goodness things were different back then! No standing about in huddles nattering instead of getting on with the work!

At weekends I used to help Dad behind the bar in the club. By this time I was seventeen years old. There was a man who used to chat me up regularly. He was a member of the club. I used to collect empty glasses from the tables. If Joe was there (that was his name) he would grab my hand and say cheekily "will you marry me next week?"

By now my plump figure had taken shape, and fined down. My measurements were at that time a curvy 37-25-37 so I suppose that wasn't bad, considering I had been a fat bespectacled child. I still wear glasses, but since my horrible childhood spectacles which I hated with a vengeance, glasses now can be a fashion statement.

Well I suppose Joe eventually got to me and we had a date at the local Picture House. I remember we went into the stalls I sat in one seat and Joe sat down a seat away from me! I remember we ate monkey nuts all through the film. I think Joe was rather shy after all so I can't say my first date with the man I was about to marry went very well.

As time went on I could tell Mum and Dad didn't want me to marry Joe. He had a disease I had never heard of: Haemophilia. This is a very serious incurable blood condition. Mum and Dad were very much against me going out with the crippled lad, as mum used to say, "you will rue the day getting mixed up with this man, never mind marry him, you will end up poor as church mice with half a dozen kids! You just want to be Florence Nightingale and nurse him you stupid girl". Well I fought against them! Mum was wrong in a lot of ways. Joe was a hard worker despite being off work a great deal due to his illness, but what did I really know, nothing of what it was going to be like!

Despite the warnings of doom and the dire consequences of what would happen if I went ahead with 'this farce', we married in September 1956 in the local church. I was by now eighteen and Joe was twenty-two. My dad who was more understanding of our feelings gave me a tot of sherry, before we left the club. He put his arms round me, and with a hug, said "come on love you'll be fine with your old dad. I loved my dad, all the upset with moving from Yorkshire and living in that horrible place in South Harrow had passed. It had been traumatic, but in the end, we had all survived, anyway they were building blocks of life. Nobody ever promised that life would always be wonderful! We walked across the road and into the church. Dad took my arm, and I walked with him down the isle and into my new life.

CHAPTER THREE

BLOOD SWEAT AND HEARTACHE

In the first few years it was very hard to cope... I had never heard of HAEMOPHILIA and the effects of this terrible disease but as the time went on I am afraid to admit Mum had been right in some of the things she had said, but not all. Life for Joe had been hard all his life up to now. He had come from a loving but poor home. He had been born with this terrible illness, how many of us would cope well in similar circumstances? I was going to make a big difference to Joe's life. I would be able to sort everything!   How wrong could I be! Joe was very frustrated at this illness, he used to get very angry at times, and as the years went by he developed a chip on his shoulder that was to become too big for either of us to carry.

He was in and out of hospital with very painful bleeds into tissue and bone.   We came back from our honeymoon on the coach with Joe on crutches! He had stepped onto a jagged rock on the beach, but you can imagine the comments we got from other people!

We started married life in rooms rented to us by Joe's boss at the time. The trouble was the man was renting the property from his landlord, and he was told off for sub-letting it to us. Very quickly we were told to move out! We searched round for somewhere else to live and found a caravan to let.

We lived in a caravan by the side of the river, but it was winter, and although the setting was lovely, try as we might we couldn't keep warm so we managed to find rooms with an elderly brother and sister. He was fine but the lady being of a delicate nature couldn't put up with the blood. Joe only had to nick himself whilst shaving to begin a nasty bleed, and as we shared the bathroom and toilet, the old lady saw more blood than she wanted to. I suppose she was frightened of something she had never experienced.

In desperation we searched the area and managed to get a cottage to let. It was situated in town. Very old and rather dilapidated, at the back there was a small room, a passage to the back, leading to a tiny kitchen where I needed to keep the light on day or night, because the tiny kitchen window let in very little light.

The sink was an old brown low-sided oblong affair. There was only one cold water tap so I had to boil the kettle when I wanted any hot water. I did manage to buy a large enamel bowl to heat the water on the old gas cooker when Andrew my first son came along. I was proud of my nappies when they were hanging on the washing line. Persil and a dolly blue bag were my washing aids. The enamel bowl also came in very useful to give Andrew a bath when he was a baby. I used to stand it in the sink. It was just the right height.

There was a scary cellar which gave me the creeps, two quite small bedrooms, the one at the back of the cottage was no bigger than a box room, you could see the stars through the broken ceiling and roof at night. We could also hear the wind and rain if it was stormy, and despite requests to mend it, nothing was ever done so you put up with it, besides we never used it. Andrew used to sleep in his cot in our bedroom.

I never did like the cellar the dark place filled me with dread! If ever I had to bring coal up, I did it as quickly as possible. The toilet to the cottage was outside in the yard. We shared the yard and the long back garden with the adjoining cottage. I loved this little house. The rent was 30 shillings a week, £1.50 in today's money. In those days you didn't complain. You just got on with it.

We hadn't been living in the cottage very long when a most frightening happening occurred. This was to be one of the most terrible times for both of us. We had been to a works dinner. Joe was employed at a local vegetable tinning factory. The boss was very good, and understood that at times my husband would be off work because of his illness. We arrived home late from the party on that fateful night. Joe was looking very pale and ill. He rushed outside to the toilet, the next thing I heard was Joe screaming out in fear for help. I rushed outside with a torch, to find him hemorrhaging badly, from his penis. I went back indoors to fetch a towel, which I put between his legs, trying to stem the flow. I got him back indoors blood everywhere. I sat him down on the only kitchen chair we had, and ran as quickly as I could to the nearest telephone, which was on the corner of the road just up the hill from the cottage. In those days, very few ordinary people had their own phone.

The doctor arrived in minutes followed by an ambulance. Joe was taken to hospital where he stayed for about ten days, he was given blood transfusions and other medication. We were to experience many such events in our early years until eventually new and more convenient procedures were developed. In between frequent visits to hospital with similar bleeds we just got on with our lives.

We found the cottage very nice to live in albeit very run down and old. We were overrun with mice. We used to sit at night and listen to the wireless, and later on when things got a little better in the purse department, we watched our black and white television. The mice as well as cockroaches used to run about the place. We put this down to living opposite a bakers shop. They sold the best cream doughnuts I have ever tasted. It was a different world back then, I remember one evening picking a little mouse up gently in my fingers, he was sitting on the corner of our fireplace, washing himself and watching the television. I must have frightened him because I had put him outside in the garden because I didn't want to kill him, but the next morning my good Samaritan act had been in vain. The little mouse was where I had left him the night before dead as mutton! He must have died instantly because he was as stiff as wood. I felt sorry for the poor little thing!

By this time I had finished work as a cleaner at the cottage hospital, the reason being that despite many protests from local people and dignitaries, the old hospital was pulled down in favour of houses. After a little searching, I managed to get a job in the main hospital in Evesham.

I had been working there for a few months on the geriatric ward, as a nursing auxiliary. I loved the job. Some of the old folk were really lovely, some, I'm afraid to say were just the opposite. I needed to tell myself regularly that one day I would be an old woman, if I lived long enough, perhaps in a similar position, to that of the patients I was looking after, and who's to say what I would be like by then? A very sobering thought!

The work was hard, but rewarding. There were times when my nose seemed to be filled with the smell of urine or excrement, and blow as I might, the offending stench refused to move from my nostrils.

The uniform for a nursing auxiliary back then was buttercup yellow dress, white apron, and cap. I loved my cap, I was also told to wear sensible black shoes and stockings. A lovely feature of the uniform was a navy and red cape, with a hood attached. I remember when I first wore this article of the uniform, I was so proud, to be seen in this creation, I was a real nurse! The red and navy cape came into its own when at Christmas I paraded with the other nurses, as we sang carols for the patients. Lanterns added to the magic, especially when it was snowing, the fresh white covering, added to the season of good will. I remember the meeting I attended when I was first given the job. Matron who seemed very straight laced at the time but who turned out to be a great help to me, warned me never to accept sweets or chocolate from the patients. I was soon to discover why! One elderly lady doubly incontinent was in the habit of rolling pieces of poo, and placing them in her fruit bowl and offering the unwary nurse or cleaner, a chocolate! I would have thought that all members of staff who cared for this lady were aware of this little trick but I do remember one of the new cleaners being caught out! Mrs Turner at the age of ninety knew exactly what she was doing, she was a wily old girl, it was evident by the glint in her eye. She was a smelly old woman, but I quite liked her. I admired her spirit and her zest for life unlike some of the patients who fed up with their lives just wanted to die.

One of the jobs I found the most difficult was laying out the dead bodies. In those days the early sixties it was still practice to pack each orifice of the dead person. I found this procedure rather disturbing at first I couldn't get rid of the idea that I was hurting the man or woman, who an hour before had been warm and alive! However, as with most things, and after a few bodies it becomes routine practice, although I must admit I sometimes shed a tear at the passing, especially if it was a dear old soul who had touched my heart in some way.

What I did find difficult at times was to leave my work at the hospital door as I left for home after an upsetting shift. If an old dear had been in tears because an expected visitor hadn't arrived, or a son or daughter had made an excuse why they couldn't come to see mum today and hadn't shown up then it got to me. I hadn't worked at the hospital very long when I was given the name Singing Canary! This was no doubt down to the fact that I was always singing around my ward, and I wore a bright yellow uniform. I loved to sing, and could be heard all over the ward. The patients seemed to like it, some would ask me to sing that song or this one. Usually they liked the old ones. Well that wasn't difficult, as I preferred some of the good old songs.

People used to say I had a decent voice back then; in fact I did used to sing on the stage at the club at weekends. In my teens and twenties I was able to reach the high notes but I was to lose my singing voice many years later in my sixties after a little heart attack. Being unaware of things to come in the future, I threw myself into my work at the hospital.

One morning I went on duty and wondered why my colleagues were smiling. I was very soon to find out why. I used to go on these daft diets, convinced I ought to lose some weight. I was by now about eleven stone. The Sister on the ward at the time used to tell me off: "you need all your strength to deal with these patients nurse, stop worrying about silly diets." I walked into the side ward expecting to see one of the old dears. Well she had passed away over night. I was met by Sister and one of the other nurses. The door to the small room was closed, I was literally chucked onto the bed, and a bowl of cold porridge, left over from breakfast was shoved into my mouth! By the time I realized what was happening I was covered with porridge, all over my uniform. They even stuffed some down the front of my bra! Sister laughing said "now tell me you are going on a diet". Well to be fair they did take me to the bathroom and give me a bath, and a change of clothes, until I got home after my shift, but looking back, it sort of happened, you had to have a joke now and again to relieve the effects of working on an old people's ward. We saw many upsetting things whilst doing such a demanding job of work.

My husband used to say that I brought the smell of the hospital home with me, complaining that my clothes smelled of stale pee, even though I left my uniform in my locker changing into my own clothes to go home in. Of course I was unable to detect the odour, after a time I became immune to the smell. Referring back to the heart attack that was waiting for me in the future, it took about a year to recover from the effects. Unfortunately I was to lose my singing voice. I could make a noise at a lower octave, but because of the breathing I could no longer reach the high notes. I have mourned the loss of my singing voice. The heart attack had left me with an enlarged heart but as they say, you can get used to anything. I was to learn this awful truth in a big way when M.S. entered my life in my thirties and continued down the path of pain and discomfort.

After a while at the hospital, despite my love for my job, I needed to get away from death, laying out bodies and everything to do with nursing old people so I started looking for something completely different. I managed to get a job in the old steam laundry taking in soiled washing and giving out clean laundry to customers who came to the door. In between times I worked on the ironing table, quite a different kind of employment to the one I was used to but it was a job, and it was only a stone's throw from the cottage. Strangely enough I liked this work. Even stranger, something happened whilst I was working there, that had it not been true, would have been disbelieved.

I was by now nineteen years old and I had been married for just over one year. I was working on my ironing table when this man called Ken who worked at the laundry as a van driver, came over to me with a photo of him and his wife's wedding. I thought how nice it was. They do say that truth is sometimes stranger than fiction. Well that is perfectly correct! What was to happen in later years was nothing but astounding in content! I will leave it there for the time being! You will understand why, later on in my book when the lovely significance of this will be apparent to you!

With Joe being ill and off work so much I didn't think it advisable to begin a family for a while anyway so I took the safe option of insisting that he used condoms. Not always the best thing for a romantic interlude, but most definitely it was the safest way. I can't say Joe was in full agreement with this, but I insisted.

Joe liked his drink and it was to become a bit of a problem even in the first year. I didn't blame him for wanting a beer, he had enough to put up with. The trouble was he used to go out with his mates leaving me at home on my own. I loved my little cottage but it could become very lonely if Joe stayed out all hours. On occasions he was known to stay out all night. Oh he sometimes asked me to go to the pub with him but it wasn't my cup of tea. Most of his pals were a good bunch, they had all grown up together mostly in the same street so I suppose it was natural that Joe wanted to carry on as he always had. However, going out boozing wasn't what I wanted, a nice meal out would have been nice but Joe was never what you might call romantic so he used to do what he had always done. Trouble was, if he drank over the proverbial eight pints, which was quite often, he turned nasty and shouted a lot. This was to put a heavy strain on our marriage and this is where the hurting love came in.

I fell hopelessly in love with a kind caring, loving man. He was a good few years older than me who showed me nothing but kindness and gentle love. He aroused in me something that couldn't be denied but the affair was doomed from the start. I couldn't leave Joe and it would have ruined the other man. I was between a rock and a very hard hurting place! I thought at the time that I would never recover from the heartbreak of the affair. We were a sickness to each other that there wasn't a cure for but in life, because of certain circumstances, things happen, and you take a road that in the end leads to heartbreak. I suppose some things you never completely get over, you just learn to live with them. It's like putting a bandage on a cut. The wound eventually heels but you are left with a scar for life. Joe punished me for the indiscretion. I would rather not say how but I didn't care any more what he did to me. Something inside me had died!! I had hurt him where most men feel it the most, in his pride! I had showed him up in front of his mates,

but it is true what they say and despite everything, you do eventually get over it. You reach a point of hopeless inevitability where you either get on with it or you don't!

If the other road had been taken, too many people would have been hurt. I couldn't have lived with that!

Many is the time I have cried tears of frustration and utter hopelessness but nevertheless, I was able to move on, albeit I was dragging the hurting debris with me for a long time.

I was to learn at a much later date many years down the line when I was in my forties, settled and accepting in my life, that sadly, the man in question had passed away a single man.   I was to suffer another heartbreaking phase of self- punishment and what ifs, once again going through mental anguish of remembering just how much we had loved each other. However, once again I was able to tuck the hurting into that special place, deep inside and get on with my life, to all intents and purposes getting on just fine.

I left the laundry and went back to the work I loved. I found another job at the hospital in our town as a nursing auxiliary where I stayed for a while. Eventually Joe and I mended a few bridges. It had to be that way for every-one's sake. Many years later Joe actually said to me "if I had treated you better back then, it wouldn't have happened." Well, I don't know whether it would, or wouldn't, but I can say, that in later years Joe and I became best mates.

When I was twenty I became pregnant with my first son Andrew. He was a dry birth, and very painful. I started labour pains on a Saturday night and he was born the following Monday. I had to stay in hospital for the two weeks before his birth and the two weeks after. The reason being, I was suffering from Toxemia. I remember being told off by the nurse in charge for laughing during exercises. All we new mums were lying flat on our beds, doing these tummy training pull-ups between your legs. It was the sight of a pair of enormous feet in the bed opposite my own that made me laugh so much. I was made to do these exercises again all on my own because of this. Actually the whole ward was in uproar! Those were the days! I had so much milk I was able to feed babies whose mums didn't have enough milk of their own. I used to look like a busty film star when I wore the glass bottles on my boobs that expressed my milk.

I brought Andrew home but the lad turned night into day, right from the first day. He slept most of the day and stayed awake most of the night. By the time my son was three months old, I was a bag of nerves. I had breast fed him for as long as I could but my milk turned to water, and I had to put him on the bottle.

At one point I was so run down I had to go to the hospital and have a large boil with a few heads lanced, I can see the kidney bowl to this day, placed under my right arm pit to collect the puss.

Andrew was to suffer repeatedly with a bad chest. The cottage was so damp that the poor little chap was a regular visitor to the local hospital. I seemed to constantly be in a fog of the coal–tar burner. Everything in the house smelled of the vapour. We all went out smelling of the stuff for ages. When he was about twelve months old, we were in for another bad time because of the Haemophilia. Andrew was crawling around on the kitchen floor. Joe had come home from work feeling ill. I had sent him to bed to rest. The next thing I heard was this awful wailing noise coming from upstairs. I don't remember climbing the stair, but I was in the bedroom, to find Joe stiff as a board halfway across the bed, his arms reaching up to the ceiling, fitting, eyes rolling in their sockets, froth pouring from his mouth.

I did no more than run back down stairs, pick Andrew up into my arms, and run round, to the people who lived up the road from us, I explained quickly, dumped the baby in my neighbour's arms, and ran to the phone box, and called the doctor. He arrived so quickly running his car right onto the pavement. The ambulance arrived shortly after. I went to hospital with Joe where I stayed as long as I could but I had to get back to my baby. Fortunately an ambulance coming back to Evesham brought me back but not before I had been told by the doctor to expect the worse, a car would be out in the night to inform me that Joe had gone, so grave was his relapse.

Apparently, and I didn't know this until Joe told me later, his push - bike had been hit by a car and he had come off and banged his head on the floor causing bleeding on the brain. He had made his way home and said nothing! Joe was stubborn like that. He said later he hadn't wanted to make a fuss but he had mentioned it to the doctor at the hospital when he came round.

Well I can tell you. That was one of the worst nights of my life. I was never passionately in love with Joe but I did love him, if that makes sense. I was worried about the outcome of this latest relapse.

I took Andrew into bed with me, and every car that went past my window I thought would be the one to tell me that Joe had gone but morning came calm and quiet. I knew without being told that Joe had come through the night. He stayed in hospital for about two weeks.

Eventually, after a lot of help from our local doctor we managed to get a Council flat on the local estate. It was a nice place, all mod-cons but I hated it. After living in town with all the hustle- bustle and shops on my doorstep, it was an event to see the baker and coal-man or the grocery van come round our street. I remember crying to Joe that I wanted to go home   He used to say, "you are home."   Well we lived on the estate for over twenty years, seven in the flat the rest in the house but it was never really home.

When Andrew was about four years old he gave me the fright of my life. He and the boy from across the road had decided it would be a good idea to take themselves to the park which was about half a mile from our house. He had been told, as always not to go off the end of the street. I was busy washing, my twin-tub washing machine wobbling about on the kitchen floor, I was saving up to buy a new one. I looked out of the window for the umpteenth time where I expected to see the boys playing but they were nowhere to be seen. I dried my hands and went downstairs to find them. I rushed across to the other boy's flat and knocked on the door. Mrs. Bradley came to the door. I had hoped against hope that the boys were playing there, but no, she didn't know where the boys were either. By now I was beginning to panic. They must have been gone for half an hour. Back then in the 1960s I don't think we worried so much about children being taken off by paedophiles but nevertheless it was frightening. It was decided that we had better call the police which we duly did! A constable arrived in his car, took a lot of details, I could feel Mrs Bradley was blaming me. She was rather stuck up in her thinking and talked rather posh. She liked to wrap her Toby up in cotton wool but she lived on a council estate the same as me. Joe used to say the woman had delusions of Grandeur.

We waited a further twenty minutes or so, by now I was standing in the middle of the green. Suddenly a police car came into our street, loud hailer blasting out " we have a child a little boy about three. Is he yours Mrs" he said looking at me.   I went towards the car, Mrs Bradley just behind me.   It was Toby, apparently he had been found on the path by a woman who lived in one of houses skirting the road, which ran past our estate. When it all came to light, there was another boy involved who lived further up the street, he and Andrew had left Toby behind because he wanted to go home. Donald (that's the other boy) and Andrew had actually walked all the way to the park! Fortunately it was the school holidays so there were plenty of children about. When the older ones with bikes got wind of my lad and Donald still missing they set off on a different route. By this time I was frantic with worry.

Joe was in hospital with another bleed so I was managing on my own.   Mrs Bradley had taken Toby indoors. I was waiting anxiously at the side of the main road when suddenly in the distance I saw the girl from the end of our street riding and waving furiously. As she came nearer, I was able to see two stubby little legs sticking out behind her, she had put Andrew on her seat and she was peddling. I don't think I had ever been so frightened. I didn't know whether to chastise or hug my boy. It was about three pm but Andrew was put in a bath, given some tea and tucked up to bed!

My younger sister Sandra had had her first child by now a girl called Lyn, and from the start the cousins hated each other. Every time they met they fought. Well it so happened that Sandra had come to visit, she lived with her family at the other side of the estate. I was baking at the time, Andrew used to love to help me (more of a hindrance really but I thought it would help him to learn to cook). I had made pastry for pies and tarts when the kids decided they wanted to make some too. I put them at opposite sides of the table gave them a piece of pastry each and some baking tins and showed them what to do. By the time they had dropped lumps of pastry on the floor a few times, rolled and needed the stuff , you can just imagine what the colour was like! They each put some mucky pastry into the tins. I gave them a blob of jam each, and popped the creations into the oven. Both kids washed their hands and went into the garden. Sandra and I went into the front room and were enjoying a cup of tea and a catch up. Neither of us saw what happened next. I went back into the kitchen to take the finished pies out of the oven. By now Lyn had come back indoors eager to see her pies. She gave a yell. "Look at my pies, they have been covered in dirt".

Andrew had sneaked in whilst Sandra and I were talking and had put a spoonful of garden dirt on his cousin's jam tart! I felt ashamed of him, and didn't quite know what to say... so I smacked his bum and sent him to bed. Andrew is 52 years old now and when I told him I was writing my autobiography, he said "don't forget to mention the dirt in the pie Mum"! I don't know why we didn't like each other back then, but we just hated each other on sight. Andrew has five children of his own from two marriages. The first failed as they sometimes do. Lyn is a Grandmother herself now. Sandra and I have had many a laugh about this!

The upstairs flat, although nice and supplying everything we needed, wasn't ideal... The old couple that lived in the flat under ours began to complain about the noise from the children. I could see their point, until one upsetting day when the old lady asked me if the boys and Joe could make less noise when going for a wee! That was the last straw!! I began to pester the council for a move, and eventually (when David was two) we were moved to a house in the next street with three bedrooms and a lovely big back garden.

Mind you we very nearly didn't move, we had taken a lot of our belongings round to the new house the evening before we actually moved in.   We had taken all our ornaments and a lot of the boys' toys. We had left a small window open at the back of the property. Bad mistake!! When we moved the next morning, all our ornaments and children's toys had been stolen! Over night.   It was probably kids, but although we called the police nothing was ever found. It made me feel sick I almost didn't want to move anymore, but it was too late, there was no going back! However later and after the police assuring us that it was children most probably and it wouldn't be a grown up thief, we settled in and eventually I felt better about the whole business. It was a lovely house and we couldn't let what a couple of kids had done spoil our change of life. We had a house, a proper house, with a lovely garden. We were going to enjoy living in it no matter what!

Life would always be a struggle never knowing when Joe would be rushed to hospital in Birmingham. But now at least we had a nice home.

One thing we did when everything was settled into its place the boys and me held hands and jumped up and down on the floor. It had been a nightmare trying to tip-toe around the flat. The boys were beginning to walk permanently on their toes because of the hassle from the flat below. I asked myself sometimes why the Council house managers thought it a good idea to put old folks in downstairs flats and families upstairs.

All I know is my life was a constant battle between Joe being rushed to hospital with another bleed, and me being worried out of my mind, or struggling to make ends meet, trying to take care of my boys. I remember back then that I would experience slight numb feelings in my fingers and occasionally, one of my legs would go to sleep, a feeling of pins and needles but I didn't pay much heed to it at the time. I just put it down to overwork.

Yes it was a struggle at times, I had never even heard of HEAMOPHILIA, never mind deal with the consequences of a heamorrhage, and looking back over those years, eighteen years old, was rather young to be dealing with the consequences of something I knew absolutely nothing about. That was my age when I had to deal with one of Joe's bleeds... so right from the first, life had been a struggle.

One of the upsetting parts of those days was the times Joe had to go into hospital with another bleed at Christmas! I used to witness twitchy curtains from neighbours' houses as the ambulance once again came to take Joe into hospital. Many's the time the boys and I stood on our doorstep and watched the vehicle leave the end of the street. To us it was the worst of times. I felt sorry for Andrew and David. In fact on one of the sad occasions David asked me angrily "why is it always my dad"? I couldn't give the lad an answer that would have made him feel any better!! I went with him in the ambulance as often as I could, but having nobody to look after my boys it wasn't always possible.

One snowy Christmas, not long after Joe had gone to hospital, a man from an organization called THE ROUND TABLE knocked on my door. He gave me a lovely looking pork pie and a box of groceries, wished me a happy Yuletide and left... I just stood and wept.

David my youngest was born almost six years after his brother... Right from the first David was a live wire, when he was only two he had toddled into his dad's greenhouse and tipped some of his dad's prize flowers upside down in their flower-pots... The thing was though, young as he was he must have realized he had done wrong and promptly put them back , unfortunately he had put them back upside down! Of course, according to his dad, it was my fault for letting him do it!!

Andrew was wonderful with him and helped me with him quite a lot, fetching nappies and other baby toiletries. As they grew up Andrew used to take his brother swimming to the local baths, he never seemed to mind that his little brother wanted to tag along. It wasn't until Andrew was about twelve, And David six, Did Andrew start complaining. "Do I have to take him everywhere Mum?" I understood my eldest boy not wanting his baby brother in tow all the time. But we worked around it.

When my children were older and both attending secondary school I had a yearning to go back to some sort of nursing. I was working part time in a local cake shop, not very inspiring, it wasn't really me. However, the cheap cakes went down very well with my boys. After a time, the cake shop closed down so I got a job at one of the local butcher's shops. The manager had advertised for a mature woman to serve behind the counter... I was by now thirty four, so I thought that would be mature enough. I applied for the job and got it. Apparently because the manager employed a couple of young men and boys he didn't want a Dolly bird to put them off their work so I fitted the bill perfectly.

I started work in the summer, and appreciated the door being permanently open. It let in a gentle breeze, which was very welcome. As time went on I had sussed out who of the customers were poor and who were the better off . It soon became apparent who the old ladies preferred to be served by! I know it was wrong but I used to put a bit of extra mince or a few sausages in the bags of the old folks I knew to be struggling. I think the boss was aware of this little misdemeanor but turned a blind eye.

I worked hard there. Polishing shelves at the back of the counter, I used to enjoy cleaning the shop window outside, I could have a chat to people as they passed by… The lads were great they treated me like mum. I was there with plasters and bandage if they cut themselves. They used to ask my advice on how to get a girl interested in them. I used to tell them to be themselves, be clean and always be polite. Don't know if it worked, but they all wanted the advice. There were three lads and I got on well with them all.

Working in the butcher's shop in the winter took on a whole different experience. The door still had to remain open even on the coldest days. Instead of a cooling breeze in the summer it was now a raging gale. Now it, didn't matter how many layers of clothing I wore, (two long vests two pairs of thick knickers trousers and jumpers), I couldn't keep warm. Touching ice-cold liver with bare hands was something else. I talked the manager into letting me have a small heater under the counter but it only helped if I was standing in front of it. Trouble was we all wanted a warm!

The toilets outside in the yard, had never seen a woman's touch, nor did they have a lock on the door, I very soon got cleaning material bleach and disinfectant, and set about bringing a pleasant place to sit when the need came. I also made certain that a lock was placed on the toilet door!

I had been working there for almost two years, when an acquaintance came into the shop to tell me there was an opening for a night care assistant at the nursing home where she worked.

I talked it over with Joe, he said "try it if you fancy it" so I did, and got a job looking after the residents of the home. I had found my niche. I loved my new job; taking care of elderly people was what I liked. I was back doing the job I loved. By now I was thirty six. The manager of the butcher's shop didn't take too kindly to me leaving but realising there was nothing he could do to stop me, gave me his best wishes.

Once again I was taking the smell of urine home with me, along with other aromas connected with an old folks home. These weren't all bad, my husband passed comments that the stink of bleach and disinfectant and cooking was even in my hair. In those days all the meals were cooked in kitchens at the home; I don't think that is the practice nowadays.

My sons Andrew and David didn't seem to detect the smell, and if they did, they never said. They just knew that Mum worked at the Old People's Home on permanent nights, and that was how it was. I suppose it must have been a bit awkward when I had to work over Christmas, but that was the way of it. The weekly rota was made out in the office and that was that. Sometimes we were able to swap shifts with another nurse but the trouble was nobody wanted to work over Christmas especially the nurses with children, so if Christmas Day came on a Thursday we'll say, and it was your shift, then you usually had to work your night shift.

On occasions my mother in law looked after David if Joe was at work and I was on an awkward shift at the nursing home. One particularly harrowing time I recall was when David was about five, he managed to cover his hair in green gloss paint whilst he was at Granny's. As I approached her house I could hear her anxious voice, " your mother will go mad when she sees this. " I walked into the house to be greeted by my mother-in-law rubbing lard into David's hair. The sight was never to be forgotten.

Apparently there had been a half full tin of green gloss paint in the back yard of the house. It had been used to paint the shed.   David and his cousin Paul who had been there earlier had found the tin, opened it and this was the result! Well I can tell you that it took more than lard to get rid of the paint, I had to use scissors to cut away most of it, although I was unable to remove some of the paint from his scalp. That unfortunately had to gradually wear off.   David was semi bald for about six weeks. He said he wasn't going to school like that!! But he did, much to his disgust. It was a lesson well learned. He didn't mess about with gloss paint after that!

My boys got into many a scrape during their young lives. Sometimes the mischief was over the top. One particular time the boys had been missing for ages, despite my warning as to what would happen if they ventured beyond the end of the street! I had called and called both of them to come in for their dinner.

After there being no response from either of them, I began to get worried... Joe by now fed up with waiting for his lunch took the car, and looked all over where they usually played. He came back to the house to see if they had come back! But no not a sign of them. They were playing with a friend so Joe went to their house to see if they could shed any light on where the boys might be. They didn't know either!! So both men set off in their own cars to widen the search. Both came back with nothing. By now I was tearing my hair out, I was thinking the worst, I think you always do! Joe had just put the car in the drive when two ragamufimins came slinking round the corner, black as the ace of spades. They had left the other boy at the end of the street. His garden backed onto ours.

Joe walked towards them, and in a voice that was far too quiet, asked "where the devil have you been, your mother and I have been very worried, your dinner has been ready for ages. Well what have you got to say for yourselves?"

David the dirtiest said in a defiant voice: "we didn't want any dinner anyway did we Andy". Joe really angry now, said to the boys, "Right then you can get to your room and bed." Both boys looked at me for support, but I looked away this time. I had been out of my mind with worry. "You heard what your Dad said." Both boys slunk past us and clambered none too quietly up to their bedroom. It was to turn out that they had been where they had been warned not to go, a mostly disused railway line!

After a while when things had become calmer, I asked Joe if I could give the boys a bath and take them a drink of milk and a biscuit. His answer was what I expected. "No Dot; they've got to learn". I sat longing to take a drink to them, but I knew Joe was right.

Later as we sat and ate our dinner, mine was choking me. There came a knock on the door. It was my brother-in- law wondering if the boys had been found. David, on hearing his favourite Uncle, shouted down the stairs, at the top of his voice... "is that you uncle Eric? Tell mum to give us some food." Well that broke the anger, and we began to titter. The next thing to happen just made me laugh out loud. David had crept downstairs and was standing by the open fridge door! Mouth full of cheese! At five years old David had a lot of spirit.

About that time we had lived in the house a few months and it was a far cry from the flat. The old couple next door, not being used to young children were a bit of a headache, always moaning about the boys making too much noise. Also they didn't like cats, and we had been to the cat rescue centre for a kitten as soon as we went to the house. We called her Tinker. She was a lovely little cat, the boys used to play with her. One day the old lady had made a meat pie for lunch. It had always been her habit to put the pie on the windowsill to cool. Well I couldn't believe what Tinker had done. The little devil had jumped up to the windowsill and grabbed hold of the meat pie. By the time I realised what was happening she had brought her booty into our out-house and was devouring it!

To my shame I never did tell Mrs Turner what had happened to her husband's dinner! Of course the boys thought the whole episode hilarious. All the poor lady found was her tin plate that had held the pie, on the floor by her back door. Tinker lived to the ripe old age of twenty years.. At the time of her death I was in the middle of an M.S. relapse. The nurse was coming to the house every day to give me injections. Tinker was on her last legs but I kept on trying to prolong her life. Tinker used to like to jump up on the draining board and drink from a running tap. She had always liked to do that. The nurse kept on every time she came, saying that the cat should be put down. As I was having my injection, Tinker jumped up to the tap and started to drink. "See" I said to the nurse, "she can still jump up?" However, a few days later I had to agree. My little cat had reached the end of the road. I had been keeping her alive just for me! She was put to sleep and I cried for her...she had been a little sweetheart and I would never forget her.

I must tell you of another trick that David pulled, it was during Christmas 1970. David was six. I had splashed out and bought some Cadbury's chocolate baubles for the Christmas tree, I couldn't really afford them but it was Christmas and the boys would love them. I was partial to a bit of good chocolate myself, and still am! We had all had our Christmas dinner. I had refused to let the boys touch the chocolate treats from the tree, until Christmas day. Andrew said "Would you like a chocolate Mum?" "Yes please", I said. I reached up to get one and to my surprise my fingers flattened the silver paper that was supposed to be covering the chocolate treat inside, I tried another. The same thing happened...

Eventually David admitted taking the silver paper from some of the chocolates very carefully taking the chocolate out and putting the silver paper back very carefully so as not to be discovered! Apparently this little bit of mischief had been done weeks before Christmas, and nobody had been any the wiser! His dad was furious with David, but eventually he got over it. My self I thought it a bit of neat work, I don't know how he managed the deceit!!

Later on when the boys were a bit older, they had gone to Badgers' Brook another place I had forbidden them to play. This place was known to flood. They had gone there in the school holidays. It had been raining quite hard for a long time, so the brook was unstable. When their dad found them they had banked the brook at one end and almost caused a heavy flood. I am afraid they both got a slap at the top of the leg from their dad for that little escapade and were sent to bed. I suppose a slap on the leg would be frowned on now but kids need discipline as well as love. That is the trouble with society these days.

Another time not to be forgotten , I had been on my nightshift at the nursing home. I had arrived home in time to get the boys off, David to school, Andrew was seventeen and in his first job. Joe had started work at his job at seven thirty. I arrived home just after eight. Andrew was old enough now to take care of his brother for half an hour. I made myself a cup of tea had a piece of toast and a couple of sleeping pills before going to bed for a few hours. I found it hard to sleep in the day time.

On this particular day I was woken from my drug induced sleep by David shouting through the letter box, I went downstairs in a fuzz. I opened the door, and what met me certainly woke me up with a start, David was sobbing, he was holding the side of his face. He came in and when I saw his cheek I was mortified.

From his ear right across his face was a deep red raised wheel. I was furious when he told me what had happened... Apparently he and another boy had been throwing a ball across the classroom whilst waiting for the teacher. David told me Mr.X came flying into the classroom grabbed him round the neck and smacked him hard across his face. David was crying while he was telling me, most unusual for him, he had always been able to stand up for himself. He was never a cry-baby. I was furious. I rang Joe at work and asked him to come home as soon as he could, I explained what had happened and that I was going round to the school at once. I rang the head master and told him I was coming to see him and asked him to get Mr. X into his office. The headmaster asked me to make an appointment with the secretary. Well! I was still under the influence of the two sleeping tablets I had taken earlier in the morning. I can tell you I was in no mood to be dictated to!

As Joe arrived home, I had thrown some clothes on and was ready for battle. I explained to the head master what had happened and that I was coming to see him NOW! and to get Mr. X into his office.

When we arrived at the school it was lunch time, we were greeted by a load of boys eager to tell us what they had seen. We were ushered into the office asked to take a seat by the head master who looked a bit peaky. Mr.X came in, walked towards me and put out his hand. I refrained from accepting, and asked him to explain why he thought it was alright to abuse my boy in such a way!

Well he kept telling me he hadn't done it when I knew damn well he had... If I hadn't believed David which I did… I had added proof from the other children. I know boys can be boisterous, and at times naughty, but this was over the top. All of a sudden I was on my feet. I brought my left arm back and clouted the lying teacher full in the face. There was uproar! The head master; surprised at what had happened said " Mrs B. Really you can't do that" but I had, and didn't it feel good, this man had hurt my boy and to be honest I was glad I had given him a smack.

A bit later when everything had calmed down, and he did finally admit that he had been a little hasty. I promised him two things, that if he ever touched my lad again the National Press would have a field day and I also promised I would not tell David that I had floored him until he left school and that would be quite a long time as David was ten years old at the time of the incident.   When we got back home I told David everything would be fine now.   Joe was also taken aback at my outburst. I sometimes caught him looking at me and smiling to himself.

I had promised this teacher, two things!! . That if he ever laid a hand on David again , the National Press would be informed. I also promised I wouldn't tell David what had happened just as long as he was a pupil at the school. David was at the time of the incident ten years old. I occasionally asked if everything was ok with this teacher, David told me he never touched him again, If we went to school parents' day or anything else connected with school this particular teacher always gave me a wide berth...Joe never quite got over my slapping the teacher in the mouth. When David left school at sixteen I told him what had happened on that day. His answer was "I thought something must have happened Mum, and you never said". His wife told me ages ago that this little story is David's party piece! He had mentioned to her that this particular teacher had always had it in for him until the day I bashed him.

After that things had changed for him.

When David was seventeen he bought a second hand scooter it was the time of MODS and ROCKERS. He and his mates were MODS I didn't like him having this bike, but he had a mind of his own and always managed to talk me round. His dad used to go mad at him. Every weekend David would take the bike to pieces in the back yard . When he put it together again there were always nuts and screws scattered about the back patio. David told his dad, who asked how he expected the bike to go properly... his answer was always the same "it will still go alright." Nobody was more relieved than me when eventually the bike was swapped for a car.

They do say that history has a habit of repeating itself. Also like mother like daughter. I must have got my slapping the teacher from my mum. I remember going back all those years to my school days when mum slapped my teacher for putting that horrible big wooden dummy in my mouth. Her smacking made life a little better for me at the time so perhaps a bit of rough justice does pay off, in some cases!!

When I was thirty six years old, I began to feel numbness here and there in different parts of my body again... The first time was when I was turning a bedridden patient, a dead finger being particularly troublesome. I mentioned this to my colleague who was helping at the other side of the bed. Her answer was" don't worry Dorothy. It's probably a touch of cramp."

Well this feeling continued at various times. A numb tongue for a little while, or a similar feeling in one leg, sometimes my hand would feel strange. I suppose I put it down to the punishing workload at times and tried to dismiss it.

However, unfortunately, the annoying dead finger, or dead somewhere else began to get to me so I went to the doctors. He asked questions, wrote down notes, and told me not to worry. He said the work I was in could be demanding, and advised me to try and take it easy, and not get stressed up but over time, this began to make me feel like a crank! Was there something wrong with me or was I imagining most of it?"

One particular evening on my way to work I remember I felt so tired I could hardly put one foot in front of the other, Joe always offered to take me to work in the car but I preferred to walk the short distance. It was a nice country stroll especially on a summer evening but this evening, it would have been better if I had stayed at home. By the time I reached the nursing home I was fit for nothing. I had been forced to rest by the side of the road, against a garden wall. I felt very weak and uncoordinated, and more tired than I had ever felt in my life. What was wrong with me?

My colleague who was on duty with me met me at the Duty Room door. Her first words to me were, "you don't look very well, you shouldn't have come in tonight" - and with no further ado she pulled two easy chairs together, making a bed, she made my lie down. Well - for once, I didn't argue, I felt too out of sorts. Fortunately, apart from Matron, and a senior nurse, who lived upstairs in the building, there were no other members of staff on duty at nights, and being as the duty room was on the ground floor, there were no other people in and out. I must say though that I felt a little guilty but my colleague -and good friend wouldn't take no for an answer.

After a really punishing week of overtime, two of the old folks passing away in the same night, the work had been hard. Plus the fact that my colleague, and I had worked ten nights on the trot, because one of the other two night staff had been on holiday. There were no extra staff employed to cover nights off, it was the same for all of us.

We had a set of fifty buzzers on a plate set on the wall of the duty room. Each one was connected to the resident's rooms. It was the job of the night staff to check all rooms every hour. We weren't allowed to use the lift after 11p m, so we had to go up and down the three flights of stairs.

Well to my shame I didn't hear one bell go off all night. I did as my friend suggested and lay on the make shift bed. The next thing I knew was that it was 7 am and I had slept all night. I awoke to the sound of early morning chores being carried out.

My friend popped her head round the door. "You're awake then, I'll bring you a cup of tea in a moment".

The next thing to happen sent me into a panic, "what ever is wrong with your face Dorothy, it's drooping down on one side?"

I couldn't move, my legs felt like lead. I tried to speak but it was all slurred and I was frightened, and the fatigue I felt was alarming. Joe was sent for and he took me home and called the doctor. He came some time later, examined me, and said in a matter of fact way.

"Well Dorothy, this could be a number of things, a slight stroke, Bells palsy, Meniere's Disease.

Then he laughed as though trying to make light of the situation, "or perhaps it's water on the brain or

even something I would like to keep under wraps for the time being."

Both Andrew and Joe were with me at the time. I don't think they could see the funny side.

The doctor advised complete bed rest for a couple of weeks. "Come and see me Dorothy after that."

I did as the doctor told me, and rested for what seemed a long time to me, what I did find upsetting was the fact that for a time I felt uncoordinated, and off balance. I didn't know where the floor was in relation to my feet, it was a very strange sensation but I did begin to feel better. The tingling and numbness went and I didn't feel so tired.

Eventually my doctor sent me to see a Neurologist consultant, at the hospital. After asking me a lot of questions and doing various tests I was sent for a lumber puncture at a hospital a few miles away. I will never forget that experience if I live to be a hundred.

I was the patient now. I was in a hospital ward with a lot of other people, the other side of the coin so to speak and I felt vulnerable. It crossed my mind, just how many times I had stood over a bedridden patient who probably had felt just as unsure as I did right now. Had I been reassuring to the old dear who found herself in this position? I hoped so.

A nurse in a green uniform came to the side of my bed holding papers.

"Now dear, I need to ask you some questions".   I looked at this woman, and tried to smile. She asked my name, my age and lots of other questions. She asked my occupation. "I'm a nursing auxiliary," I said weakly, trying to get her on side. The green nurse gave me an unimpressed smile, "are you dear- how nice?"

She wrote a few things down on her important looking paper. She pulled the curtains around my bed, and gave me a hospital gown to put on. " Wait there dear, Doctor will be with you shortly."   I took a deep breath. Where else would I be?

I heard the familiar sound of trolley wheels trundling down the ward; I looked to where the noise was coming from. Suddenly the flowered curtain was pulled to one side and two nurses, and a doctor all wearing masks poked their heads round.   The rather rotund nurse asked me in a kind voice to turn onto my side and pull my legs as far as I could up to my chest. Both nurses held me in that position, one pulling at my legs.

I heard the doctor say "just a prick in your back dear, keep perfectly still". The next thing to occur was probably to cause the most pain I had ever felt in my life, up to that point. I felt the needle pierce my back...

As the excruciating hot pain shot down both legs, I let out an almighty scream. I remember one nurse looked across at the other with real concern in her eyes. I don't think that was supposed to happen. I should have had an injection to numb the area. I am as sure as I can be that I was not given it! I was then told to lie to on my back for twelve hours and stay as still as I could.

Looking back over that time, the thing that has given me many a smile was what happened at lunchtime on that horrible day. As I gazed up at the hospital ceiling wondering amongst other things how long since it had been painted and how dingy it looked (as if it really mattered to me- one way, or the other),

a young trainee nurse brought me a knife and fork and placed it on the table that straddled my bed.

Very soon I could smell the meal cooking; the same nurse who had brought the knife and fork came along with another nurse pushing the food trolley. I could smell lovely fish and chips.

By this time I was about five hours into the prone position, and rather fed up with myself.

A plate of fish and chips would be lovely. Well it wasn't to be! Oh I was brought a plate of fish-chips and peas, by the same trainee nurse who placed it on the tray way above my head, smiled and walked away.

I attempted to feed my self from my prone position, but after many tries with my fork to spear a piece of battered cod, with peas and bits of fish and chips all over my bed, I gave up. The best of it was, the same nurse came back later and asked me: "didn't you like your dinner dear?" I remember telling her that, had I been able to reach it I would have been able to eat it! I just might have enjoyed it!

I am not sure that particular nurse had what it takes to be a caring Florence Nightingale for her skills at noticing what was right in front of her nose, left a lot to be desired!

I was discharged later in the week and told to see my own Doctor. When I did make an appointment I never expected the news that the doctor gave me. I walked into his consulting room, sat down and asked what the verdict was. The doctor sat across from me behind his polished desk. He was very quiet.

Then he said: "are you sure you want to know Dorothy?" I tried to sound brave, although I was feeling anything but. I said in a voice that sounded like it was coming from my boots,

"if I had cancer I would rather know." He looked at me for a moment and reaching into his desk drawer, he pulled out a large sheet of paper.

On the top of the paper I read my name and in big letters the words DISSEMINATED SCLEROSIS, He said it was the American name for Multiple Sclerosis, I have learned since that DISSEMINATED is an old name for the disease but either way, it wasn't something I wanted to be told I was suffering from.

Trying to sound braver than I felt, I asked what it meant in terms of life. I had come across this devastating disease in my job, and never once did I associate my illness with this horrible life-changing affliction.

Mind you I had only come across this illness in the latter stages, so how could I possibly associate my early symptoms with the couple of old ladies in the ward, bed ridden, and needing so much help. I had never come across Multiple Sclerosis in the first stages before.

This kindly man looked me full in the face. He asked again "Are you quite sure you want to know my dear?" I nodded back to him.

"Yes I must know what I am fighting." He removed his glasses as if that would make the telling of bad news easier.

"Well my dear, with the knowledge we have at the moment it is about twenty-five years at best and five at worst.

I remember I just sat there. This wasn't real. It wasn't happening to me! I would soon be going back on night duty; I couldn't have this horrible illness. I was too busy; I had my family to take care of.

I had jobs to do; besides Joe wasn't well, in and out of hospital. It was too cruel that both of us had a terrible illness. This couldn't be happening!!

I walked out of the doctor's room and went to my Mum and Dad's bungalow tears streaming down my face, and was met by Dad's outstretched arms, and his comforting voice,

 "Come on lass tell your old dad what's happened."

I can recall to this day my parents' tears as they tried to take the news in.

When I told Joe he was sympathetic to the problem, but he was made of strong stuff, his own illness had made him so. He was a fighter, life for him had been hard, he did have a chip on his shoulder, and who could blame him, but at times it was difficult for me to live with.

However, from the start Joe was very good, and it must have been difficult for him. After all he had had to put up with his own illness all his life. To have to take on mine as well must have felt rather like an extra burden he could have done without but having said that, I know he helped me when I was feeling sorry for myself in the early days. His attitude was, there isn't much you can do about it. You will just have to live with it. Well of course he was right. After all we live till we die. How we get there largely depends on us.

By now we had been married for almost twenty years, so hurts of the past where somewhat dimmed. Mind you, every little argument we may have had always brought with it an undercurrent of what had gone before. For example remarks like, "I bet you wish you'd gone off with him" were just under the surface but I had grown a thicker skin and just answered him, "well I didn't did I?"

Inevitably, and I guessed it would happen, I was informed that I could no longer be employed at the Home. Matron was very kind, but told me: "you need to be fit and strong to do this work, so unfortunately we must terminate your employment with us" so at the age of thirty seven, I felt I had been thrown on the scrap heap. My illness took another backward turn.

Well of course there was no way I was fit to work, and for the next four months, I seemed to crawl around, not knowing quite what was happening to me. I wasn't sure where the floor was in relation to where I was putting my feet, that was a bit scary, also my trunk seemed numb, I found it easier to lie on my stomach than sit on my bottom which at times felt like a block of wood.

However, I think one of the worst sensations at that time was in my private parts. It felt very uncomfortable and I lost any inclination of wanting to be touched there. I became very depressed, and try as I might I felt very scared, and also very alone, although I had my family. Looking back I suppose I was pretty pathetic. I felt so depressed, and my imagination went into overdrive.

I felt I was in a deep pit of misery, unable to claw my way out because the sides of the pit were too slippery... this was a very scary feeling. For a time I was given anti depressant drugs, I just couldn't come to terms with a brain illness, and the 'why me?' syndrome ruled my life. I must have been a pain in the backside back then. I voluntarily attended a Psychiatric Clinic for a few weeks; it wasn't my cup of tea. I felt ashamed of having a mental illness. The doctor was a bit impersonal. He asked me lots of questions and wrote my answers on a notebook. When the questioning became too personal, too searching I stopped going. My private and personal life was none of his business, so I thought.

I didn't really know what M.S. was. I researched the illness and although I couldn't understand some of the big words associated with the disease, I had a pretty good idea what the implications were. I learned that the word Sclerosis meant scars, and multiple meant many, and that wherever a scar appeared on the brain, that was where the attack had been.

I remember with dread, the first MRI Scan I had on my brain, it was horrible. I hate the contraption with a vengeance but I realize this procedure has to be done, but I still have a dread of that noisy machine. I am a bit claustrophobic - and having my head enclosed in the contraption is horrible. As time went on I was to experience this quite a few times.

Joe had mellowed over the years, drink not being such an issue, and he was very supportive, and tried to tell me that it didn't matter that I could no longer go out to work "you'll have enough to do at home", and when I mentioned money he said, "we will manage."

Well, we did manage. We had been able to save a little when we were both in fulltime work but it wasn't a great deal. There were just a few pounds saved here and there in a post office savings account. I was able to get a disability pension, after being told by the M.S. Society to apply for one, as I was entitled to help of this kind... My doctor advised me to join the M.S. Society, as I would meet other sufferers. Well I did join, but to my shame I didn't stay for long; seeing people in wheelchairs used to upset me, that wasn't going to be me. I suppose for a long time I was in denial and even tried one or two part time jobs, but I had to eventually give in.

I remember when I was unable to walk very well, owing to an early relapse I found it safer to crawl around on the, floor. Well I thought to myself: you can't fall off the floor can you? This used to upset Joe, especially when one day he came home from work to find me crawling about the sitting room. He devised a way to get me to the toilet or to the sink to have a wash. He would hold me round the waist, put my feet on his and walk me backwards. It was a bit scary but he managed it.

Looking back to when I was first diagnosed and using the wheelchair, my boys used to argue who was going to push me. I remember one particular time when we went to DEVON for a few days, during my first few months of having the illness. Joe said the sea air would do me good and pick me up a bit. I remember vividly being pushed along the front in my carriage by two over enthusiastic sons. I gripped the sides of the chair and I was reminded of an old film I had seen (THE KEYSTONE KOPS), I was quite safe, Joe saw to that, but even so it was a bit hairy.

On the whole, my boys took the news pretty well. I felt for them though. A dad with HEAMOPHILIA, and now me with MULTIPLE SCLEROSIS! This was a bit much to take on board for two young lads. I carried on suffering little relapses and recovering again.

However, the worst was yet to come. One day out of the blue, I felt a pain in my jaw that almost floored me. A sharp stabbing sensation that I had never experienced before- and it terrified me. This was the start of a life long battle with M.S. into the TRIGEMINAL NERVES both sides of my jaw causing intense Neuralgia... Nothing on earth could ever feel as bad as this. At its worst the pain hammers my jaw, so much so that on two occasions I have passed out onto the concrete floor of our little patio. I fell backwards both times, and was rushed to hospital with a split head.

My doctor put me on drugs by the names of CARBANAZAPINE and GABAPENTIN, The latter didn't seem to do much good, but I still take the first drug today when my enemy strikes again.
The side affects to this tablet are horrendous. They seem to affect my off balance more. They make me

very tired, I am unable to function properly and they make me depressed, but, they are the only thing that takes away the pain in my jaw so it is a love –hate relationship I have with the drugs. I hate what they do to me, but I am completely dependent on them for adequate pain relief.

For some reason both sides of my jaw are a favourite place for my M.S. to attack. If I try to tell you the intensity of the pain at its worst then I would fall short but my consultant told me that at its height, it is the worst pain known to man. He had known strong men weep, and in some cases take their lives because they couldn't stand the pain. Therefore, you will understand the sheer severity of the hell when this pain strikes. Mind you I don't know why this dear man would think that bit of information could help me? As time passed I was to suffer bouts of BILATERAL TRIGEMINAL NEURALGIA and up to date, I am 73 now, I have had five operations to the right and left sides of my jaw. I pray this will not occur again but I just try to stay focused on what's good.   As long as my jaw stays numb, then it should be ok!

Going back a bit, before M.S. entered my life, we were almost like other families, and we managed.

My wages had gone a long way to helping with the housekeeping. Joe- because of his illness spent a lot of time either off work or in hospital, so money was always tight. The boys needed things, school uniforms, a treat now and again. I used to feel very sorry when their peers seemed to have things that my boys were denied. One Christmas when Andrew was about nine years old he had wanted a two wheeled bike. I didn't think at that time we would be able to afford one but we somehow managed to get him one.

Christmas morning arrived. Joe had managed to conceal the bike in his shed. He brought the bike into the house and into the room. I will never forget the look of surprise on my boy's face. Andrew just stood tears in his eyes transfixed looking at his new bike. I had to choke back a few tears of my own.

I remember once when we managed a few days at Weston-Super –Mare during the school holidays. Joe had been in hospital again, and I had a few days off work, so we decided on a few days by the sea.

We had taken a small self -catering flat on the front. The boys aged about twelve and six respectively were walking along before us full of excitement. We were looking for a café to have a meal. Andrew, looking at the menu in a café window shouted out with enthusiasm:

"I'll have a pork chop and chips." His dad from behind answered, not too unkindly:

"you won't son, you'll have egg and chips and like it, we haven't got pork chop money."

From that day many years ago, I have never forgotten that request for a pork chop from my boy, and the refusal by his dad, I can still see the look on Andrew's face . I really felt for my boy, it seemed to signify our struggle, a struggle that was to become more evident as the years continued...

We spent many times at the hospital where Joe had to go for blood transfusions. On one momentous occasion, when Joe was supposed to go to hospital, and he was too ill to drive himself there, Andrew at the age of fifteen, drove his dad all the way there. Joe had to stay in for treatment. The car was left in the hospital car park (there wasn't any parking fee in those days). Andrew came back by bus. Joe came home in his car when he was better. I admire my brave son, but we could have been in trouble if the police had seen what had happened. Andrew has since told me that had his dad's car not been automatic then he wouldn't have been able to do it. He said an automatic is a doddle to drive! I just think my son was very brave.

That was a very worrying time, it sent my M.S. into overdrive for a while. However, as the years passed by and medicine developed, Joe was able to manage without the need for travelling thirty miles to have treatment, blood products became easier to administer at home. We were both shown how to give intravenous transfusions, and so began a much easier phase of managing Joe's illness. I do remember though with dread, when I first began to administer the transfusions, as I tried to get the needle into the chosen vein, it would sometimes collapse, and I had to try another, perhaps in Joe's ankle. The kitchen at times, resembled a blood bath, it was a bit hair-raising but we always managed.

When Joe was fifty seven he became very ill with a growth. He spent many weeks at home on a made up bed down stairs because he could no longer manage the stairs. Nurses, from the hospital, came to bathe him. This was a waste of their precious time, because his response to them giving him a bath was always: 'Dot will do it", his name for me.   Well I did bath him just as long as I was able, but it had to come to an end, when I could no longer get him out of the bath, it was a strip wash in the bathroom from then on.

Unfortunately it soon became obvious Joe needed to go to hospital, where he stayed for about six weeks. I was able to visit every day owing to the fact that Andrew my eldest son drove me the thirty miles to the hospital. The journey was punishing and took its toll on me but I was thankful to my boy.

We had a dog at the time called Ben a lovely border collie cross. We all adored him. Mum took care of him while I visited the hospital. She was supportive, as much as she could be. She lived alone now as Dad had passed away some years before.

When the medical people couldn't do any more for Joe, he was taken to a hospice. The place was lovely. They really catered for Joe's every need. They even let me take Ben to see him, unfortunately the dog didn't seem to know his master in that different environment, and Joe asked me sadly not to take Ben any more. That upset me a lot, it was as if Ben knew his Master was dying and he couldn't cope with it, or, perhaps it was the different smells that upset the dog.

Well for whatever reason that was the last time Joe was to see his beloved Ben... I put together a collage of family photos and pinned them to a large board and we took it to the hospice, this seemed to please Joe. I spent the last traumatic week of his life there in the hospice with him. My mum looked after Ben the dog for the whole time I was staying in the hospice, I used to phone her every day, and she would beg me to come home for a rest, but I couldn't, I had to stay with Joe.

There was a Catholic Priest at the hospice that used to visit Joe on a regular basis. We are not catholic but I blessed this nice man for being there for Joe.

Towards the end just before Joe went into a coma he asked me if I could see this young man by the side of his bed dressed all in white. Joe said to me, "he's not one of the family but he is helping me."

The priest explained to me that the image Joe could see was his own angel...All I know is that to Joe, this young lad was helping him and that made me feel better!

David my youngest son was living and working in Yorkshire, he was to become a successful business man in the future. He came to see his dad as often as he could, in fact he was able to visit while his dad was still conscious, the day before he went into a coma. I was informed by a nurse who was caring for Joe, that he wouldn't last much longer and to expect his death soon. I rang Sandra and explained the situation. She dropped everything and came to the hospice at once. I was so glad to see her so when the time was drawing near the time, two nurses came to sit at the opposite side of Joe's bed. I had been telling Joe a few jokes. I was also trying to sing his favourite song to him, in my now feeble voice for they do say that the hearing is the last thing to go. One of the nurses leaned over to me and said. "you must tell him to go Dorothy, it's his time." so I said to Joe, in a shaky voice. "Come on love, your mum's calling, you had better go and see what she wants".

Joe died with my arms round him at that precise moment, with his eldest son, and my sister by his side, in that peaceful hospice at the age of fifty eight. He was much too young to lose his life. He had struggled until the end and lost the battle.

As he drew his last breath a tear squeezed from his eye and trickled down his cheek. I was to recall that touching end many times in the near future. Andrew and I both came home broken. My sister was very upset, myself, physically and emotionally drained.

I was by this time 54 years old. Joe's death had been traumatic; we had been married for thirty-six years, it hadn't always been easy, in fact sometimes I hadn't known which way to turn. Although my boys were good and supportive after their father's death, coming to see me when they could, they had by now their own families.

I felt very alone in my little house. I had Ben my dog, he missed his master, as well, we used to cuddle up together, and I cried a lot. I remember the lonely nights. My nerves began to trouble me. I was sometimes afraid to be on my own, very glad of Ben's company.

We also had a rescue cat, we called him SHA, He was a beautiful pure white Persian cat, hence the name; he had the fattest, fluffiest tail I had ever seen. Well that was to grow to maturity later. When we first had him he was only five weeks old, and fitted in the palm of my hand not old enough to leave his mum, but unfortunately she was a very old cat, and had rejected him. Joe didn't want a cat, but I could see that this kitten needed a home, and nobody else seemed interested in the little scrap so I pleaded with Joe, until he gave in. I worried at first as to how old Ben would react to this bundle of mischief, but I needn't have. They soon found out the pecking order, and got on very well.

After Joe's death home wasn't home any more. I didn't like cooking for myself. I couldn't be bothered. I used to enjoy baking and cooking nice meals but for one I just didn't like it. I remember, I hated to go to bed alone, so I would sit up until two or three in the morning, either watching some rubbish on the television for company, or listening to a relaxation tape a friend had given me, but I soon got fed up with listening to songbirds, or the gentle waves lapping the shore.

Later on a close friend came to stay with me at nights, I was able to focus on her arrival and cook a meal for both of us... This helped me a great deal but I was to suffer another relapse. This was inevitable, I suppose. Stress is one of the worst things for M.S. My Mum, who lived about five minutes away, and other members of the family and friends did their best to help me cope

but at times I thought I would have another mental and
M.S. break-down.

CHAPTER FOUR

A NEW BEGINNING

I loved our house, a semi in town, but far enough away to be out of earshot from the sound of traffic. David by now was 18 years old. Andrew had left home a few years before to get married. David had worked in one of the local food factories but he was never really happy there. He asked me one day if I could think of anything exciting he could do. Well I had heard of a place called a KIBBUTZ. This was a place in ISRAEL, a commune, where everyone helped each other. I had heard about this place when I was working in hospital. David was so interested that he went the next day to the library to find out all he could. Well to cut a long story short, David and his best friend Nick went to get the information they needed and we saw them off on the train for their first part of the journey.

Before he had left David who loves music and owned a little record player, said to me that he had left his favourite record on the deck ,with the arm ready to flick on when he came back. He hugged me and said

"it will be like I've never been away Mum". I never did tell my boy how much I missed him and that for the first two weeks after he had gone to ISRAEL, I couldn't even go to his room without crying my eyes out.   The boys were in ISRAEL for almost one year.   Sometimes I was to wish I had never suggested it at the time. The trouble was, and I hadn't realized it, there was war in BERUT. David used to write home every week telling us of all the wonderful things he saw, and was doing. He never did tell us until he came home just how close they were to the war... Most of his letters told of cleaning out the camels, or going swimming in the Dead Sea, he said he visited King Herod's Palace, and the place where Jesus was born. Anyway the boys came home in good shape. The experience seemed to open David up, filling him with the need to explore further afield. From then on he began to journey abroad on far away holidays.   I learned a valuable lesson that every parent needs to know and that is, you only keep your children by letting them go!

Joe had loved his garden; he had been retired from work owing to his ill health for a number of years and with his disability pension and mine, we managed quite well financially. We had even managed a week in CORFU where our youngest David almost twenty years old had been working as a Jack of all trades, master of none in a little place called the BUTTERFLY BAR. He had been working there for about one year. Looking back on that holiday, it was magic. Joe really enjoyed that time abroad and so did I, it was lovely to spend time on that lovely island. David would go on to be a very successful business- man in my beloved Yorkshire. David had gone back to my roots, which meant now and again I could go back home. He employs several staff for his business and travels all over the world in his job.

The holiday came out of the blue. Fortunately, I was in another remission feeling quite well. David rang home regularly and on the last phone call, he had asked me to send him some clean clothes through the post. His dad piped up, "tell Dave we will bring him some clothes by plane" and that is just what happened. We went flight only and stayed with our son once again, in his accommodation. The Villa was basic, but we loved every moment of that holiday. It wasn't long after that lovely magical time that Joe became very ill.

I was to recall that lovely time in CORFU a lot when I was by myself. I was so glad that we had been able to enjoy that special time on that beautiful island again with our son.

I can't say I was living after Joe passed away, it was more like existing, and I went through the motions, but I could never tell anyone just how scared and vulnerable I felt. Would anyone understand the absolute aloneness I was enduring? My boys were very good, and by this time I had my first two grandchildren, this was a comfort, but I was sad and I felt rather like a fish out of water. I had relied on Joe for so much. A lot of, what ifs? began to plague my mind. For instance, what would happen to me now? Perhaps I would end up in a home! I was pretty pathetic looking back but being alone after all these years was rather daunting to say the least.

Well eighteen months into my widowhood, things were about to change for me in a big way.

I was in town shopping one day when I saw an acquaintance of mine. She stopped me and told me I didn't look very well. As we chatted she invited me to her church the following Sunday evening. Well I thought; it can't make me feel any worse than I do now…so when Sunday came I took my walking stick, and strolled down the road. The church was only a stone's throw away, it hadn't always been a church, it used to be part of the school my boys attended. To tell the truth, I thought it had been turned into a scout hut.

After the school had closed it didn't look like a church at all.

I walked into the ELIM PENTECOSTAL CHURCH…and into my new life. I felt rather shy. I was going somewhere on my own that I had never been before. I walked in and immediately noticed my friend. She beckoned to me and asked me to sit down next to her. It soon became apparent that she had told people about me, and soon a lady joined us. My friend introduced her. This lady was to feature a lot in my life during the next few years.

The service began and as I listened to the hymns and the Pastor speaking, I knew this was what I wanted.
After the service the Pastor asked me if I would like to talk to anyone. I said 'yes', and soon the lady I had met earlier came to me, and took me into a room at the back of the church.
As I began to speak, I felt a weight begin to lift from my shoulders, then the tears came, deep, sobbing tears that had been waiting for release for such a long time. The Pastor gave me a little booklet called Journey into life, I took it home, and read every word, and when I came to a prayer, which asked if you wanted to accept

Jesus into your life, I said it and accepted. Once again the tears flowed, I wept and wept quietly to myself. And when at last the weeping stopped I felt completely empty, and more peaceful than I had felt for a long time. I can't say I felt anything Religious, no banging drums or trumpets blowing but I did however feel changed.

I continued to go to church every Sunday evening. The congregation really helped me. I experienced a feeling of comradeship and love. These people were genuine and I felt at home. Up to this point I still had my singing voice. The heart attack was to come later. I loved to belt out the hymns and choruses and on occasion as time went on I was asked to do a solo.

Now something strange was to happen, some said it was all part of the jigsaw puzzle of life. I prefer to think it was part of God's plan. I had been going to church for about five weeks, when on this particular Sunday evening I noticed this man who I knew from long ago when I worked in the old Steam laundry. I hadn't seen him before in church. It turned out that he had been a member for a long time, and because of The Gulf War, which was being fought at the time, and his occupation now being with the Civil Service, he had been at work every day, for a number of weeks.   It also turned out that all at church had been worried about his welfare. Ken, (that's his name,) had lost his wife to illness about a year before I lost Joe, and he seemed to be going down and down.

Well to cut a long story short, we seemed to click, and to the amusement of all our friends we started going out together... I suppose you will have realized that Ken is the same man who forty odd yeas ago had brought his and his wife's wedding photo to show me where I was working on the ironing table at the local laundry.   The old building has been long gone to be replaced by a garage and a super-market.

My boys were a little concerned, and David, living and working with his own business in Yorkshire, rang me one day, and asked bluntly "who is this man Mother?" David had always been very protective of me. Andrew wasn't so worried; he lives close to me about a mile away, so had already met Ken.

I was able to assure David that once he met Ken he would understand my feelings, and I was correct. David and Andrew soon got to be very fond of their Step Dad, and he them.   Ken and his first wife didn't have children but now Ken has seven grandchildren, and they all love him.

Ken and I fell deeply in love and Pastor married us to the delight of all in church.

The wedding reception was a wonderful occasion. I was so proud to be Mrs Dorothy M Mitchell.

My family and friends who up to that point hadn't met Ken soon warmed to this unassuming man,

that was seventeen years ago. I moved into Ken's house after we married. It was just down the road from my own house so the area was the same... BEN and SHA moved home before I did, Ken looked after them whilst my son Andrew and my friend Mavis helped me to clear my house, getting it ready to put on the market.

Unfortunately Ben only lived for another year, and died in the place he had made his own, by the side of Ken's armchair. For quite a while SHA spent a lot of time just sitting in old Ben's place. SHA died at the age of twelve. Mr. Lewis our vet put her to sleep on a soft towel on my draining board as KEN and I stroked her, another upsetting time, but if you love animals which we both do then you have to get used to losing them, hard as it may be to come to terms with...

Soon after that, both of us being dog lovers, we decided to give another dog a home. We went to the rescue centre and fell in love with this border collie pup. He was all arms and legs and about ten months old.

He had a scar on his head, just over his eye, but he was to bring us such joy. We called him BEN in memory of my first dog. Ken and I used to take him on walks together at first, but as my M.S. became more of a nuisance my long walks up Apple tree lane had to come to an end. I occasionally used to go in the car and enjoy the country view whilst Ken and the dog went on their walk.

He unfortunately passed away three years ago, we had had him for twelve years and his passing almost broke our hearts. He had been our baby, a lovely intelligent daft as they come dog! We thought we would never get over Ben's passing.

Andrew Came to visit soon after Ben had died. He found Ken and I sobbing.

"You can't go on like this", he said, "you need another dog." At first we said we couldn't. It had been too upsetting to lose another friend, that's what our pets are to us, friends but God said to us "you can."

Well with no further ado he took us to the rescue centre. We saw and fell in love with Evie, a terrier, collie cross. Apparently she had been in the rescue centre for a few months because nobody wanted her for being too old ! .. Ok so she isn't young but then neither are we.   She is adorable and her coming to live with us, mended two broken hearts.   We don't know how long we will have her, but she will be loved, as were our other pets.   We feel sure that BEN would have loved this sweet little dog.

A strange and wonderful thing happened when Ken took Evie to the park for the first time. One of the dog walkers, who owned the dog that had befriended Ben years ago, took to Evie straight away. Apparently Zebedy, that's the dogs name, had missed Ben and had been off his food; well whether he could smell Ben on Evie, we will never know but Evie and Zebedy are best pals, the owner of Zebedy said it was strange because his dog had never made friends with any other dogs apart from Ben and Evie!

We never know why some things are so. Perhaps a larger force than us knows exactly why things work out for the best...

Much has happened during these wonderful years. Our Church is very important to both of us.

When we had been married for about two years, Poetry came into my life. I found it quite easy to put words together in poems, and to my joy, Ken said to me one day, after reading some poetry in our local paper written by a man who lived not far away, "why don't you send one of your poems into the paper?"

At first I refused, thinking that my efforts weren't worth printing. Well Ken kept on encouraging me so I sent my first poem in to the editor, and to my complete surprise, it was, accepted. Can you understand my joy when opening the paper the following week; there was my poem, my first poem ever, was entitled OUR BEN!

Well that was to be the first of over a hundred the local paper printed. I was to go on with my poetry and had my first book of my poems self published. I went on to be recognized as far away as Bermuda. A lady wrote to me from there telling me how much she enjoyed my poems.

I don't know to this day how my poetry book got to that far away place.

I was picked up by a small publisher by the name of POETRY CHURCH who published quite a lot of my work. Also two small poetry publishers called RUBIES IN THE DARKNESS, and SILVER WINGS in CALIFORNIA publish my poetry so you can say that my poems have touched a lot of people. I personally feel that this latent gift of writing is a gift from God. It must be, coming so late in my life.

Ken has supported me all the way. He is an uncomplicated lovely man, giving encouragement every step of the way. Unfortunately Ken has some illness problems namely Arthritis of the lower spine and Angina. He suffers greatly from back pain, but we look after each other. We say jokingly that God knew exactly what he was doing when he put us together the reason being nobody else would have us. In his younger days Ken had been very involved with St John Ambulance. He had reached the esteemed rank of Divisional Superintendent for the whole area. He was made an Officer Brother of the Venerable Order of the Hospital of St John of Jerusalem in 1972, and retired after forty-three years service. Ken was a bit shy of me writing this but I think it deserves a mention! Ken has been my rock since we met again after all these years, and hopefully I am his.

During this time, change affected all aspects of my life. I have bouts of M.S. but I try to always keep on top of it. Also, if I am not careful, depression will raise its horrible head and try to attack me. It still does. Sometimes I feel the threat of a new anxiety trying to get me but I just keep holding on to my Faith in THE LORD and Ken and my family.   On occasion, I feel a tear threatening. Memories from the past hurts come to visit but I think we all feel like crying sometimes. The pressures of life now are so removed from the life we used to take for granted.

My M.S. was rearing its ugly head again. I was now being attacked by the cruel enemy called BILATERAL TRIGEMINAL NEURALGIA. It is bad enough having the pain on one side of my jaw, but both sides is a bit much. I am frightened of this pain; I hate this pain with a vengeance.
It robs me of so much... The constant worry as to when it will 'get me' again wears me down. It's a constant threat, even when I am at my best. Since my last two

operations on both sides of my jaw my mouth and parts of my face are numb. Ken says it doesn't stop me from talking though!!

However, I do find this latent gift of writing such a boon. I can sit at my P C in my office,
(my little bedroom really) and get away from the mundane. I find that concentrating on my latest book enables me to focus my thoughts, on something other than my illness.

I realize that now and then I have to go into hospital for another op on my jaw, one side or the other. I think the worst thing about this confounded illness is that I never know when it will strike, and that is
Pretty scary!!

Another frightening episode happened about three years after my marriage to Ken.
I wasn't feeling very well, couldn't put my finger on what was wrong, all I know is that I felt quite poorly.
I felt very tired. My eyes felt funny. I remember vividly getting up from my bed, and having to get straight onto the settee downstairs owing to a variety of horrible things going on that I couldn't control.

There is a lovely Magnolia Tree in our back garden. My husband tells me a lovely story of how this Majestic Tree came to be there. It goes something like this:

"My Dad planted it when it was just a baby", 'something for you to remember me by when I'm dead and gone,' he had said.

My husband told me this story with a tear in his eye when I first came to live in this house.

He said that the Magnolia was only three feet tall when first planted over forty years ago. It now stands taller than the house and must be thirty-five foot in height. At the time of one of my relapses it was in full leaf. It is a really beautiful tree. The settee is positioned opposite the window. As I looked out...the leaves on the tree, instead of being sort of round in shape, and swaying gently, seemed to my eyes spiky and jagged in movement. The next thing I noticed was that the dark green of the leaves looked nondescript. Then I noticed my red slippers weren't red but a washed out dirty beige pink. I was very scared, I told Ken who called the doctor immediately, telling the receptionist what was wrong.

The doctor arrived within the hour; he took me to the dark room under our stairs. He examined my eyes. He looked worried and told Ken he would be getting in touch with a consultant in the field at once and that he should be ready to get me to the hospital in a couple of days.

Well he hadn't left the house half an hour when he rang back, to tell Ken to get me to hospital right away. He had been in touch with the hospital and they had said to get me there as soon as possible. I arrived in a fit of panic, what was wrong now?

Well it turned out to be an M.S. attack into my eyes which was to last about six weeks. They didn't keep me in hospital thank goodness and after lots of T L C from Ken I recovered my colour sight, in about six weeks. We used to make light of the situation. Ken would ask me what a certain colour of a dress or some other pretty article on the T V was. He would point out something and ask me what colour it was. To me, purple was beige and other shades weren't what they should be. Eventually everything returned to normal, and I was over another relapse.

Unfortunately there isn't much I can do about it. I sometimes feel like running up to the top of a big hill and screaming and screaming my head off, but for one thing, I would never make the climb and another I would probably be taken away and placed in a Home for the Bewildered. Joking apart, I sometimes remember the gnarled hands creeping round the door and the slippery sided pit when my nerves were upset again... it was a quite a time ago now, but I still remember the fear.

From poetry I went on to write children's books, I had a couple self published and they were well accepted. I managed to interest a Literary Agent; he began to send my work to children's book publishers. This brought limited to average success.

I then went onto writing novels, and to my joy my literary agent managed to interest CHIPMUNKA PUBLISHING with my first book called HOLLYBECK, a period novel about life lived among the very rich, and the intermingling with the working class. They have since published four more of my novels, entitled IT DOESN'T RULE ME, a fact-based fiction, and ONE FOR SORROW TWO FOR JOY followed by THE GARDEN

GNOME'S SECRET and THE SECRET OF WILLERBY GRANGE.

My latest work to be accepted is my new novel entitled TO LEAD US HOME. This latest book is in memory of our BEN. It will stand as a testament to how much this faithful dog meant to Ken and me.

He had had a bad start in his life, before he came to us. I suppose you can say it is a story of many a poor dog who has to go through trials before he or she, finds a good home to call their own!

I feel so blessed that people seem to like my work. I feel especially blessed that Ken and I are together.

I have a lovely family, two sons, who are very supportive! I have two lovely Daughters in–Law, seven Grandchildren and Evie our little dog. I love them all. I have some wonderful friends, one in particular who has helped, and guided me. He is a fellow writer. His name is Martin .P. Buckley. Taking me to hospital on occasion when I am in a relapse, friends like this are worth more than gold. Unfortunately for Ken, because of his own severe back pain he finds the journey to Bristol Hospital too painful.

I will carry on with my writing just as long as I can... I can't allow M.S. or the associated nervous issues to rule my life. I can't and I won't!   My next adventure will be continuing to write books for children. I really enjoy the magic. I can transport myself into realms of wonder and delight where anything can happen!

Who knows, perhaps battling with others' illnesses, and problems, and your own, for most of your life, makes you a stronger person, growing you into the man or woman you are now. All I know is...I have up to now lived a bit of a flowery life, smiling and hurting my way through! However, I also know with absolute truth that as long as I have a life I will embrace all it throws at me and who knows perhaps one day I will write a best seller.

P.S. I really want to thank Jason Pegler, and the lovely team at CHIPMUNKA for persuading me to write my autobiography. Personally I don't think I am important enough to warrant a book about me! I found some of it upsetting, but on the other hand it has enabled me to see certain aspects of my life in a different way. So yes! Putting my life down on paper has done me good. I hope you enjoyed the read.

DOROTHY M MITCHELL

www.ingramcontent.com/pod-product-compliance
Lightning Source LLC
Chambersburg PA
CBHW031208270326
41931CB00006B/467